Nurses and their patients: informing practice through psychodynamic insights

Other Health & Social Care books from M&K include:

Research Issues in Health and Social Care
ISBN: 978-1-905539-20-8 · 2009

Perspectives on Death & Dying
ISBN: 978-1-905539-21-5 · 2009

Identification and Treatment of Alcohol Dependency
ISBN: 978-1-905539-16-1 · 2008

Inter-professional Approaches to Young Fathers
ISBN: 978-1-905539-29-1 · 2008

The Clinician's Guide to Chronic Disease Management for
Long Term Conditions: A cognitive-behavioural approach
ISBN: 978-1-905539-15-4 · 2008

The ECG Workbook
ISBN: 978-1-905539-14-7 · 2008

Routine Blood Results Explained 2/e
ISBN: 978-1-905539-38-3 · 2007

Improving Patient Outcomes
ISBN: 978-1-905539-06-2 · 2007

The Management of COPD in Primary and Secondary Care
ISBN: 978-1-905539-28-4 · 2007

Pre-Teen and Teenage Pregnancy: A twenty-first century
reality
ISBN: 978-1-905539-11-6 · 2007

Issues in Heart Failure Nursing
ISBN: 978-1-905539-00-0 · 2006

Nurses and their patients
informing practice through
psychodynamic insights

Edited by

Louise de Raeve
Mic Rafferty
Mary Paget

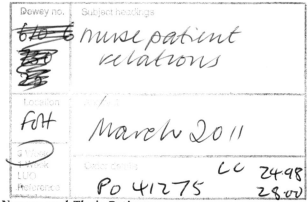

Nurses and Their Patients:
Informing practice through psychodynamic insights
Louise de Raeve

ISBN: 978-1-905539-31-4

First published 2009

British Library Cataloguing in Publication Data
A catalogue record for this book is available from the British Library

Notice
Clinical practice and medical knowledge constantly evolve. Standard safety precautions must be followed, but, as knowledge is broadened by research, changes in practice, treatment and drug therapy may become necessary or appropriate. Readers must check the most current product information provided by the manufacturer of each drug to be administered and verify the dosages and correct administration, as well as contraindications. It is the responsibility of the practitioner, utilising the experience and knowledge of the patient, to determine dosages and the best treatment for each individual patient. Any brands mentioned in this book are as examples only and are not endorsed by the Publisher. Neither the publisher nor the authors assume any liability for any injury and/or damage to persons or property arising from this publication.

The Publisher
To contact M&K Publishing write to:
M&K Update Ltd · The Old Bakery · St. John's Street
Keswick · Cumbria CA12 5AS
Tel: 01768 773030 · Fax: 01768 781099
publishing@mkupdate.co.uk
www.mkupdate.co.uk

Designed and typeset in 11pt Usherwood Book by Mary Blood
Printed in England by Ferguson Print, Keswick

Contents

List of contributors

Alyson Charnock RMN, Dip.PP, BSc (Hons), MSc.

Alyson began her nurse training in 1981, qualifying as an RMN in 1985. She has an extensive background in mental health nursing, working within all areas of mental health, especially acute psychiatry. She undertook a number of practice development, audit and quality assurance roles before gaining her current post as a Clinical Governance Manager in Abertawe and Bro Morgannwg NHS Trust. Her current role involves nursing specific clinical governance issues, having several articles published about the implications of governance in nursing. Alyson has a specialist practitioner degree in community psychiatric nursing (BSc Hons) and completed her Masters Degree in Nursing at Swansea University in 2007.

Heather Davies D. Nurs. Sci., MSc, DMS, PG Cert. (HEd), RGN, RM.

Heather has considerable experience in management, education, research and clinically in the field of cancer and palliative care. She has undertaken much development work in the field of clinical supervision and clinical effectiveness. Research interests include suffering, stress and coping, management and development of the nurse patient relationship.

Louise de Raeve PhD. Pg.Dip, Cassel Cert. in Psychological and Family Centred Nursing. RGN (previously)

Louise trained as a registered general nurse in the early 1970s, having first obtained a degree in philosophy. After a five-year period nursing at the Cassel Hospital, she moved into nurse education, becoming the Macmillan Lecturer in Nursing Ethics at Swansea University. Louise has now retired from teaching, in order to develop her private practice as a psychoanalytic psychotherapist.

Mary Isaac RGN, MSc.

Mary qualified as an RGN in 1977 in Neath General Hospital and then worked there initially as a Staff Nurse, then a Sister in Theatre Recovery and later in the Intensive Therapy Unit. In 1995, she moved to Prince Philip Hospital, Llanelli as a Senior Nurse. In

2004, she gained the position of Directorate Nurse for Surgery in the Carmarthenshire NHS Trust while at the same time studying successfully for the MSc in Nursing.

Alun Jones PhD, MSc.

Alun is an adult psychotherapist at the North Wales NHS Trust, Department of Psychological Therapies, Wrexham. Alun has published and presented research at conferences, both nationally and internationally. Alun has clinical experience developing liaison psychiatry services in the 1980s, including planning psychological nursing interventions for people with physical illness. Areas of specialist practice have included psychotherapy with the seriously ill, the dying and bereaved, working with people with cancer, HIV and AIDS and cystic fibrosis in different medical settings. Alun is currently a clinical supervisor to trainee psychotherapists of different disciplines, including medicine. Until recently, he was also a research supervisor to undergraduate and post-graduate programmes, including doctoral research studies. He has had experience working as an external and internal examiner to undergraduate, MA, MSc, MPhil and PhD research programmes. Together with a colleague, Alun is currently involved with the management of a qualitative research study in Wales, concerning mental health service users' and health professionals' experiences of shame. This study, which employs focus groups, has attracted a NHS Trust research and development grant.

Lois Jones RGN, Dip Nur., RHV.

Lois qualified as a RGN in 1984, working then at Morriston hospital till training as a Health Visitor in 1992. As a Health Visitor, Lois worked in a busy multiethnic city medical practice until struck down by encephalitis in 2000. Lois worked then as a training coordinator for health visitors and school nurses. Lois retired from health visiting in 2005, and now works as a nursing support worker with the children's disability team in Swansea.

Wendy Kennedy MSc, BN (Hons), RN.

After qualifying as a Nurse in 1999, Wendy worked as an anaesthetic nurse for five years, acting in the last year as a practice development nurse. For the last four years, Wendy has been employed as the Transfusion Practitioner in ABMU NHS Trust, more recently undertaking a Divisional Clinical Governance role as well her Transfusion work. Wendy has had several publications in peer reviewed journals which reflects her interest in developing nursing knowledge and delivering quality patient care. She enjoys the challenges of working for the NHS and has an avid interest in how politics influence nursing.

Mary Paget RGN, Dip N (Wales), BSc Nursing (Wales), MSc, PGCtHE.

Mary qualified as a general nurse in 1981 and worked in a range of clinical areas before settling in Acute Medicine for Older people in 1984, working as both staff nurse and ward sister in this area. She moved into nurse education in 1998 and is now working as a Lecturer in Adult Nursing in the School of Health Science at Swansea University. Mary has a particular interest in the impact on older people of living with chronic conditions such as stroke and cardiac disease.

Mic Rafferty RGN, RMN, MN, Cassel Cert. in Psychological and Family Centred Nursing, PgDip (FE).

Mic has a clinical background primarily in mental health therapeutic communities for children, adolescents and families in the UK and USA. In nurse education since 1985, he developed educational programmes about dementia care, full reflective practice and clinical supervision, with a research and publication record in these areas. He has held management responsibilities for both clinical practice and staff development at the School of Health Science, Swansea University. Mic retired from full-time work in 2005 and currently works as a part-time lecturer in clinical supervision.

Grace Sansom MSc, BSc, RMN, RGN.

Grace's nursing career spans nearly 30 years during which time she has worked in many varied roles across numerous specialities, and with many teams, including both general and psychiatric nursing, in both primary and secondary settings. This provided the foundation for taking on corporate nursing roles, fulfilling strategic agendas, focusing on quality and clinical governance aspects of care. Her known love of mental health nursing has recently resulted in the opportunity to become Assistant Head of Nursing for this service, to assist with the current Trust merger. Grace has undertaken research at BSc and MSc levels, authoring a number of mental health specific articles.

Sally Williams BN (Hons), MSc, Registered Paediatric Nurse.

Sally's clinical background is in general medical paediatrics, high dependency and neonatal nursing. She has worked for the School of Health Science in Swansea University as a nurse tutor in Child Health since 2004, and in 2008 commenced a three-year secondment as a research nurse for CRC Cymru. Sally has an interest in neonatal nursing and meeting the complex care needs of children.

Foreword

In June 2008, just before this book went to press, the UK Health Secretary Alan Johnson announced that nurses are to be scored on their compassion for patients as part of a new drive to improve the NHS. The compassion index, he said, would be compiled by health regulators using surveys of patients' views while in hospital, including feedback about the attitude of staff. 'Nurses to be rated on their smiling and compassion skills in new government drive' said the *Mail on Sunday* (18 June 2008), adding that Mr Johnson: 'believes putting a smile on the face of nurses and encouraging empathetic care is as important to recovery as the skill of doctors in the operating theatre.'

This approach to the work of nurses is of interest in a number of ways. First, it is self-evidently true that the way nurses relate to patients will affect the patients' emotional wellbeing. Patients are, by definition, usually ill and often dependent in some way for the duration of the illness. It is this that makes them so particularly susceptible to being affected by those on whom they depend. Secondly, this insight is hardly new; indeed Louise de Raeve in Chapter 1 below points out that as long ago as 1972 nurse researchers were identifying serious problems in nurse–patient relationships which had a detrimental effect on patients. Thirdly, there is ample research which elucidates the psycho-physiological pathways whereby emotional state can affect the physical processes of disease, resistance to disease and recovery, not only the patient's emotional response to these processes. Thus we can be sure that even if the journalistic weighting cannot be evaluated (empathic care is *as important* to recovery as the skill of doctors in the operating theatre), psychological care, even of surgical patients, is *important* to recovery.

But, as de Raeve says of the early nursing research: 'The trouble … is that while they indicated serious problems in nurse–patient relationships, with the suggestion that something needed to change, they were thin on theory and hence on any substantial explanatory story which might have helped lead to a solution. At best they indicated some need for change in nurse education and at worst, they induced a sense of guilty helplessness in nurses who recognised themselves in such accounts, did not wish to behave this way and yet found that they did. The educative response is valuable but inadequate in isolation, because it fails to grasp the power of what is taking place.' (Ch1 – pages 13–14) The same is true of Mr Johnson's plans and the tabloid trumpeting of them. In relating to patients, nurses must often relate to: people who are terrified, people who are furious at what is happening to them and want to blame someone for something, people in complete or partial denial of their illness, people who are incontinent of their bodily excretions and need these cleaning up in a tactful and sensitive way and people who have lost their minds. This is to mention just a few of the conditions of the people for whom nurses are expected to smile and give empathic care. And they must do this even when the problems of the patients in some way mirror those of the nurse or her loved ones, in the past or present. How could this be humanly possible?

As this book explains, since nurses are humans with their own feelings, it is only humanly possible if attention is paid, by nurses themselves and by those who support them, to the effects on nurses of these relationships with those who depend on them. The automatic, and largely unconscious, response of many of us when faced with stressful or distressful stimuli – whether to what is happening to us, to what we are witnessing happening to another person or to the way that other person is relating to us as a result of that person's own stress – is to try and find some way to moderate the strong feelings we might otherwise experience. Often we need to do this to keep functioning. In human relating much of the associated emotion occurs below the threshold of conscious awareness, especially when the emotions involved are negative, and often professionally unacceptable, such as distress, fear, disgust or even hatred.

A theory that has the possibility of helping to make sense of the ways patients and nurses behave in stressful situations is psycho-analytic theory, the theory of unconscious functioning. But the theory alone will not help; education in how the unconscious works will not help nurses, really, any more than education about the psychological care of patients. Both of course *will* help give the nurse a framework and discipline with which to manage her practice. But in order to have a chance of becoming more aware of feelings and responses occurring below the threshold of awareness, of processing and making sense of those feelings and of possibly then moderating or changing their responses, nurses need time which is set aside on a regular basis, a skilled and understanding senior colleague and, ideally, also a group of non-judgemental peers.

This book offers theory and examples of people trying to use it – nurses reflecting on, and trying to make sense of, experiences with the help of psychoanalytic theory. It also offers some accounts of practice through the model of clinical supervision. I hope reading the book will inspire nurses to feel that the endeavour of reflecting on relationships with patients could be a worthwhile one which might be instituted much more widely than it is at present. And I hope those with the power to administer a 'compassion index' might gain some understanding of what is needed if they really hope for positive change.

Julia Fabricius
Psychoanalyst
(Member of the British Psychoanalytical Society)

Introduction

This book belongs to a context wider than nursing, where different authors have written about the way psychoanalytic thought can be usefully used to illuminate the work of health care practitioners who are not themselves psychotherapists or psycho-analysts (Obholzer and Zagier Roberts, 1994, Hinshelwood and Skogstad, 2000, Goldie, 2005). This suggests that psychoanalytic thought is fertile territory for new ideas to aid thinking about health care. Transferring such ideas, however, from their original context to more general use has to be done mindfully, for the obvious reason that the contexts are vastly different. For instance, many psychoanalytic psychotherapists work in such a way as to deliberately reveal very little of themselves. This enables a study of phenomena such as 'transference' and 'counter-transference'. Nurses, however, share quite a lot of themselves with their patients in the course of their daily work.

This means that whilst ideas like 'transference' and 'counter-transference' may be helpful ways of thinking about nurse–patient encounters, their analysis is inevitably 'muddied' by the ordinary conversational way that nurses relate. Another important difference is that the patient in therapy has signed up for something called 'therapy' or 'analysis'. The patient in a general hospital, on the other hand has signed up for no such thing. Therefore, any interpretation by nurses of the unconscious meaning of a patient's behaviour is unlikely to be confirmed or disconfirmed through dialogue with the patient. This means that such thoughts must remain tentative and speculative.

In the psychoanalytic/psychotherapeutic setting, interpreta-tions are used to help the patient to change. In the settings described in this book, such understandings are used to help nurses make better sense of their relationships with patients, survive the distress of their work and achieve more depth of understanding of their nursing role. Ultimately, the justification for using ideas out of their original context has to be that it increases the possibilities for human creativity, kindness and tolerance.

In addition to the tradition of using psychoanalytic thought to assist health care practitioners generally, another, smaller tradition has arisen, aiming to influence nursing care specifically. This has not been limited to the psychiatric nursing setting (Dartington, 1993; Fabricius, 1991, 1995). Other publications that capture some of this work include Barnes (1968) about the work of the Cassel Hospital (a psychoanalytically informed, therapeutic community) and Barnes *et al.* (1998) about the application of psychosocial nursing principles. That the authors of this current book have an interest in this approach should come as no surprise when it is learnt that two of us (de Raeve and Rafferty) worked in the 1970s and 1980s at the Cassel Hospital. Doreen Weddell, the first matron of this hospital developed the idea of 'psychosocial nursing' with her team of staff. This influenced people such as Anna Dartington (an ex-Cassel nurse) who for many years ran courses at the Tavistock Institute for Human Relations, for nurses. Sadly, she died recently.

The discerning reader may notice that many references in this book are common to many of the chapters. The explanation for this is that this book grew out of a Master's level module on Psychodynamic Perspectives of Nursing and Midwifery. Most of the students doing this eleven-week course had no previous knowledge of this way of thinking. The case-study section of this book is formed from the assignments that these students submitted, although these have been extensively re-worked for this publication. The resulting chapters demonstrate how these ideas can be used to make sense of the complex, everyday experience of nursing. The powerful explanatory capacity of these contributions offer nurses a significant way of explaining why they feel the way they do. Such understanding can lead to insights, which inform responses, thereby enhancing the capacity to practice with integrity (de Raeve, 1998). The fresh, and lively way in which these authors have approached the task of translating psychodynamic ideas and applying them to their practice, provides a means by which they can be easily grasped by other nurses to inform their practice.

This book is therefore intended as a resource for experienced and inexperienced nurses from across the professional spectrum, wishing to think more deeply about their practice in a psychodynamic way. The editors have a long-standing interest in, and commitment to, the value of these ideas to inform patient care and to protect the thinking capacity and emotional well-being of the nurse. Ultimately, such ideas inform what can be considered to be the proper and healthy nature of health care systems.

There is relatively little literature on the relevance of psychodynamic thinking for nurses and nursing. A literature search produced the following list: Kenney (2001), Terry (1997) and Barnes *et al.* (1998). None of these take the same approach as this book, which offers perspectives arising from the practice of ordinary nurses with little previous exposure to such ideas.

The focus in this book is upon significant psychosocial events in nursing and how these can be understood through a psychodynamic perspective. The themes concern ordinary, rather than pathological development and behaviour in the life cycle. The structure of the book supports the core chapters written by those who did the psychodynamic module. There are three sections: 1. Theoretical, 2. Case-study, 3. The wider context.

Theoretical section

Theoretical section

This part of the book consists of four chapters, which provide an overview of key theoretical ideas that preoccupy the authors of the case-study chapters. Inevitably, this analysis is selective and no attempt is made to give a comprehensive overview of psychodynamic theory in this book. Rather, the aim is to show how such ideas when applied to health care, help us to make better sense of:

- making relationships, attachment and separation
- the experience of illness and loss
- the ways we manage anxiety.

Some of the specific theoretical ideas considered include: the nature of the unconscious, the nature of the parent–child relationship (good-enough parenting), attachment theory, object relations, the meaning of illness and loss, defence mechanisms (individual and social) and projective mechanisms including transference and counter-transference. The ideas derive from the work of people such as: Melanie Klein, Donald Winnicott, Eric Bowlby, Mary Ainsworth, Colin Murray Parkes, Isabel Menzies Lyth and others. Behind all these people stands Sigmund Freud, the father of psychoanalytic thought.

Nurses and their patients

Case studies

Case studies

This section contains the seven core chapters. These stories have been grouped to capture the primary themes of each. To begin with there are three chapters which address the theme of attachment:

- Lois Jones writes about her personal experience of serious illness and her search for an attachment figure.
- Mary Isaac explores the significance of a daughter's presence at the bedside of her elderly mother and the way the sister in charge of the ward understood this need.
- Sally Williams uses an account of her care of a dying child to consider the complex meaning of attachment and the importance of play in this relationship. Sally also introduces the ideas of transference and counter-transference

These are followed by two chapters that also explore attachment but, in addition, introduce the perspective of transitional objects and transitional phenomena:

- Grace Sansom defends an interpretation of the significance of a baby doll to the well-being of a woman with dementia. The intuitive understanding of this is enhanced by appeal to the theory of transitional objects.
- Wendy Kennedy reflects upon her interactions with patients in the pre-operative environment of the anaesthetic room, using three different encounters, one of which includes a ward nurse.

The two final chapters in this section explore projective mechanisms and either overtly or implicitly, transference and counter-transference:

- Mary Paget writes about the wife of a dying man who accuses her of attempting to murder her husband, via the use of a syringe driver. Mary attempts to make sense of this by understanding the relationships of everybody involved and their history.
- Alyson Charnock as a mental health nurse, describes an agonising situation concerning the suicide of a patient and her sense of burden when dealing with the responses of the mother.

Each chapter is followed by a brief commentary written by the editors, which attempts to summarise the key points, draw attention to some of the more implicit issues and suggest the wider implications for individual nurses and health care systems.

The wider context: research and supervision

The wider context

Three chapters are included in this section. The theoretical ideas explored in Sections one and two are re-visited with a consideration of how these ideas may be further used to inform practice. The first chapter by Heather Davies gives an extensive review of the research background that supports a psychodynamic way of thinking and more specifically, its application to nursing. Clearly in a world where CBT (Cognitive Behavioural Therapy) is a dominant voice and supported by research evidence, it behoves those of other persuasions to either produce similar evidence or, if this cannot be done for conceptual as well as practical reasons, to articulate clearly why this is so. It is not the editors' intention to imply that the psychodynamic perspective is better than CBT, only that in a realm as complicated as the mind, where positions taken may ultimately reflect different values, irrespective of research evidence, there needs to be diversity, rather than hegemony of thought.

In the chapter which follows, Alun Jones presents an overview of his research project, investigating the impact of clinical supervision on a small group of palliative care nurses. The last chapter, by Mic Rafferty, considers how clinical supervision may help nurses think in a psychodynamic way about their work and it offers a model derived from the work of Winnicott (Rafferty 2000) to make sense of the process of supervision.

In the chapters that follow all patients', relatives' and other members of staff's names have been changed, to protect confidentiality.

References

Barnes, E. ed. (1968). *Psychosocial Nursing: Studies from the Cassel Hospital*, London: Tavistock Publications.

Barnes, E., Griffiths, P., Ord, J. and Wells, D. eds. (1998). *Face to Face with Distress: The Professional Use of Self in Psychosocial Care*, Oxford: Butterworth Heinemann.

Dartington, A. (1993). 'Where angels fear to tread: idealism, despondency and inhibition in thought in hospital nursing.' Winnicott Studies 7 (Spring): 21–41.

de Raeve, L. (1998). 'Maintaining integrity through clinical supervision.' *Nursing Ethics* 5(6): 486–96.

Fabricius, J. (1991). 'Running on the spot or can nursing really change?' *Psychoanalytic Psychotherapy* 5 (2): 97–108.

Fabricius, J. (1995). 'Psychoanalytic understanding and nursing: a supervisory workshop with nurse tutors.' *Psychoanalytic Psychotherapy* 9 (1): 17–29.

Goldie, L. (2005). *Psychotherapy and the Treatment of Cancer Patients: Bearing Cancer in Mind*, London: Routledge.

Hinshelwood, R.D. and Skogstad, W. eds. (2000). *Observing Organisations: Anxiety, Defence and Culture in Health Care*. London: Routledge.

Kenney, J.W. (2001). *Philosophical and Theoretical Perspectives for Advanced Nursing Practice*, Boston: Jones and Bartlett.

Obholzer, A. and Zagier Roberts, V. eds. (1994). *The Unconscious at Work: Individual and Organizational Stress in the Human Services*. London: Routledge.

Rafferty, M.A. (2000). 'A conceptual model for clinical supervision in nursing and health visiting based upon Winnicott's (1960) theory of the parent-infant relationship.' *Journal of Psychiatric and Mental Health Nursing* 7 (2): 153–61.

Terry, P. (1997). *Working with the Elderly and their Carers: A Psychodynamic Approach*, Houndmills, Basingstoke: Palgrave

Part I

Theory

Chapter 1
The nature of the unconscious
Louise de Raeve

Introduction

Nurses are well used to caring for unconscious patients and they may be observant of the fact that some unconscious patients sometimes give indications of mental life, such as dreaming. Indeed on regaining consciousness, patients will sometimes recall that, while they were aware of things happening to them and around them, they thought they were somewhere other than a hospital, on board a ship for example (personal communication). It is not, however, this idea of unconsciousness that is the focus of this chapter. Instead I aim to present some aspects of a theory of the mind which has a specific conception of 'the unconscious'. This theory of mind was created by Sigmund Freud and his associates in the early days of the development of psychoanalysis, towards the end of the nineteenth century and the beginning of the twentieth century (Freud 2001). As Laplanche and Pontalis state: 'If Freud's discovery had to be summed up in a single word, that word would without doubt have to be "unconscious"' (Laplanche and Pontalis, 1988, p. 474). Despite its long history, this view of the mind, while disputed by some, has many adherents. Eric Kandel, who won the 2000 Nobel Laureate in Physiology or Medicine stated that 'psychoanalysis still represents the most coherent and intellectually satisfying view of the mind' (Kandel 1999). In what follows in this chapter, I hope to be able to demonstrate how such ideas may usefully illuminate nurse–patient relationships, although it may take the content of the whole book to demonstrate how this knowledge can also enhance the opportunity that nurses have to nurse well.

Freud (2001) spoke about 'conscious', 'pre-conscious' and 'unconscious' aspects of the mind. What is conscious is all the thoughts and feelings that we have, that we are aware of. The 'pre-conscious' is just below the surface, it contains things we might be about to become aware of and dreaming may feature here. The 'unconscious' is a surmised part of mental life that we are not able to be aware of directly. Such descriptions tend to make these aspects of the mind sound as if they are entities which have a geographical location. This would be to misunderstand that primarily, they are metaphors and hypotheses that are trying to first describe and then to explain our mental life. Having a mind at all is dependent upon having a brain and a body in which it can be located. Current ideas would locate the basis of the 'unconscious' in the right hemisphere of the brain and the conscious mind in the left hemisphere (Mollon, 2000, p. 63, citing Schore, 1993) but this is not the same as saying the mind equals the brain; it is a different sort of 'thing' and actually not a 'thing' at all. Failing to distinguish this would lead to what Ryle called a category mistake (Ryle, 1963). For the purpose of this chapter, it is more useful to think of the 'unconscious' as a dynamic force in the mind, which sometimes enhances and sometimes undermines conscious mental life. By definition, it is unknowable in its totality but rather as a jet leaves a trail in the sky, the 'unconscious' may leave evidence of its presence: evidence which can then be interpreted.

Mollon (2000, p. 5) suggests that the idea of unconscious motivation 'is an inference that provides an explanation for the gaps and distortions in our consciousness'. One such gap would be the distinction that can sometimes occur between what we consciously intended to do or say and what we actually end up doing or saying. This gap can be amusing or embarrassing, depending on the circumstances, but it is always baffling until the unconscious symbolism of what has taken place can be grasped. Sometimes this is not far from our conscious awareness and, as Mollon suggests, it may be best to think of gradations of consciousness, rather than of an absolute, impermeable distinction between what is conscious and unconscious. A colleague provided this example of a slip of the tongue: 'Cynical supervision' instead of 'clinical supervision'. One might say this is a mistake with no meaning but if it were the case that the speaker was cynical about the benefits of supervision, one might conclude that this had been unconsciously revealed by the slip of the tongue. If one finds it slightly amusing, the question arises as to why! Supervision provokes mixed feelings in people and such humour works by revealing what may hitherto have been covert. We laugh in recognition.

Another illustration of unconscious activity is 'forgetting'. This can be understood as an 'active process which usually serves some [unconscious] personal purpose' (McGhie, 1979, p. 145).

> ... I had an argument with a colleague during which I said something which, unknown to me, both hurt and annoyed my friend. A few days later I asked to borrow a book which he had at home. Although he prided himself upon an excellent memory he nevertheless forgot to bring the book on three consecutive mornings (McGhie, 1979, p. 146).

He goes on to observe that 'A similar explanation is often applicable when we forget appointments with people whom we dislike or to whom we feel hostile' (McGhie, 1979, p. 146). One can see from these illustrations that unconscious processes have a tendency to break through unbidden into conscious mental life. In the previous examples, enactments (slips of the tongue, forgetting etc.) can also be understood as unconscious communications. We can experience these 'breakthroughs' as amusing, embarrassing, frightening, baffling, illuminating and so on, depending on the circumstances. What they have in common is that their expression bypasses ordinary conscious thought and it is only later, upon reflection, that we may 'catch-up with ourselves', as it were.

Mollon (2000) gives a helpful analogy of his own to try and describe what the relationship might be between the conscious and unconscious areas of the mind:

> Consciousness could be compared to what is visible on a computer screen. Other information could be accessed readily by scrolling down the document or switching to a different 'window'. This would be analogous to the conscious and the preconscious parts of the mind. However, some files on the computer may be less easily explored. They may have been encrypted or 'zipped', or they may require a password or are in other ways rendered 'access

denied'. Some may also have been corrupted, so that information is scrambled and thereby rendered incomprehensible. (Mollon 2000, pp.8–9, citing Freud 1923)

Freud would not have been familiar with computers, as he died long before their arrival in the public domain but the metaphor of something being 'encrypted' or 'zipped' or with 'access denied' is to try and convey the inaccessibility of the unconscious to our conscious mind. It was Freud's view that the unconscious is formed of repressed material, impressions and experiences that have been expelled from consciousness. Some of what is expelled may be simply obsolete but some consists of experiences that would be too disturbing to recall in their entirety. Everybody would have these experiences, not just those people who have had very traumatic childhoods. This is because what counts as disturbing to an infant may be to do with inner, rather than outer reality, or to do with the uniqueness of the weave between the two, for any given individual.

This idea of dynamic, unconscious mental life was not popular with those who wished to retain a view that the human adult was largely in charge of his/her own life. In the free will versus determinism debate, it weighs in heavily on the side of determinism, or at least it appears to. Interestingly, a therapeutic goal of psychoanalysis would be to bring the unconscious mind into better communication with the conscious self, so that there is greater opportunity for interplay between these two aspects of mind and thus an enhancement of individual creativity, imagination and free will. Seen this way, psychoanalysis is committed to individual liberation.

The social and cultural impact of there being 'conscious' and 'unconscious' aspects of the mind has been far reaching. Expressionism and Surrealism in fine art can be seen as related to a culture where there is an interest in 'the unconscious' and this influence has also permeated theatre, where plays like Peter Shaffer's (2006) 'Equus' (originally published in 1973) make explicit reference to unconscious motivation and symbolism. To bring this influence closer to health care, consider how common it is to talk about 'denial' when somebody who is recently bereaved seems to behave partially or totally as if they were not. Yet this is an idea of an unconscious defence (nobody decides to deny, it just happens) against intolerable levels of anxiety and emotional pain, in this case, the death of a loved one. One could not talk of 'denial' without a conception of the unconscious underpinning it. Such denial is protective but also worrying to friends of the bereaved if it goes on too long, since a person using that defence is impaired in their ability to adapt to reality (there has been a death). Complete denial in such circumstances is rare but most of us will have encountered partial denial in ourselves and others in such circumstances. It is also possible to help someone move from this position to a greater grasp of the reality but not by pointing out the irrationality of their perception of events, since to do so would imply a failure to grasp that this is an unconscious process. Only by bearing with such a person how intolerably painful their situation feels, might one slowly be able to help them to face the reality that has befallen them.

Relevance to nursing

Relevance to nursing

Working with death and bereavement is a common occurrence for nurses and it is not surprising that several of the case study chapters, which follow this section, focus on this theme. A broader provenance for such ideas, however, and more specifically, for the idea of unconscious phenomena, lies in the illumination they can offer to help explain ordinary, as well as difficult nurse–patient interactions in any nursing context.

It may be remembered that in the 1970s and 1980s, when nursing research was in its infancy but being developed by a few feisty pioneers, several uncomfortable studies emerged which examined nurse–patient interactions: Felicity Stockwell (1972) for instance, with her research on the 'Unpopular Patient'; Jill Macleod Clark (1981) with her work which explored how nurses 'block' communication from patients. The trouble with these studies is that while they indicated serious problems in nurse–patient relationships, with the suggestion that something needed to change, they were thin on theory and hence on any substantial explanatory story which might have helped lead to a solution. At best they indicated some need for change in nurse education and at worst, they induced a sense of guilty helplessness in nurses, who recognised themselves in such accounts, did not wish to behave

Nurses and their patients

this way and yet found that they did. The educative response is valuable but inadequate in isolation, because it fails to grasp the power of what is taking place. This 'gap' between what nurses consciously want to see themselves doing and the reality of what they find themselves doing is, I believe, helpfully bridged by the idea of the unconscious. To assume that one can master unconscious forces by education is delusional, since it assumes that primitive impulses (such as love, hate, fear, lust) can be checked and mastered by appeal to rational argument. In fact, a purely educative approach is likely to broaden the gap between the nurse's vision of an ideal nurse-self and the reality of the nurse she discovers herself to be in practice. Fairbairn and Mead (1990) refer to this sense of dissonance as a 'a loss of innocence'. If nursing as an institution offers no way forward to help to narrow this gap, nurses cannot be blamed for trying to desensitise themselves from perceiving it. It may be simply too painful to do otherwise.

Preceding the era of Stockwell's and Macleod Clark's research, Isabel Menzies Lyth (1988) wrote her seminal paper: 'The functioning of social systems as a defense against anxiety', the first version of which appeared in 1959. Whilst this research and ensuing papers contributed to ensuring Menzies Lyth's fame as a psychoanalytical social scientist, it seemed to leave mainstream nursing largely untouched. We couldn't seem to hear what she had to say, partly I think because we did not understand it and partly because we were frightened that we were being criticised and found wanting. However, in my reading of this paper, there is much that is compassionate and insightful about both the unconscious worlds of nurses and their patients and how these may interact. Menzies Lyth points out that nursing is very difficult work:

> Patients and relatives have very complicated feelings towards the hospital, which are expressed particularly and most directly to nurses, and often puzzle and distress them. Patients and relatives show appreciation, gratitude, affection, respect; a touching relief that the hospital copes; helpfulness and concern for nurses in their difficult task. But patients often resent their dependence; accept grudgingly the discipline imposed by treatment and hospital routine; envy nurses their health and skills; are demanding, possessive and jealous. Patients, like nurses, find strong

libidinal and erotic feelings stimulated by nursing care, and sometimes behave in ways that increase the nurses' difficulties: for example by unnecessary physical exposure. Relatives may also be demanding and critical, the more so because they resent the feeling that hospitalisation implies inadequacies in themselves. They envy nurses their skill and jealously resent the nurse's intimate contact with 'their' patient (Menzies Lyth, 1988, p. 48).

Some of these feelings and reactions will be consciously expressed and consciously perceived and understood by others but they may also be defended against unconsciously, because of their disturbing quality. Such feelings may then emerge in distorted and unexpected ways which can puzzle and disturb other people. For instance, a patient's relative may find fault with the nurses because of feelings of inadequacy and guilt on his/her part. The nurses may see nothing in their own care of the patient that would give reasonable cause for the relative's annoyance. Such nurses may become puzzled and flustered and, then feeling unjustly accused, become angry. It is likely to be helpful to the nurses at this point, if they have some understanding of what might be going on, because they then have more responses in their repertoire than simply an angry reaction or the stifling of anger. The options might include tolerating the accusations because of knowing that sharing the patient can be very difficult for relatives, or it might be openly acknowledged that today the relative really seems to need to find fault with the nurses, or someone might comment that it must be very hard being the relative who until now did all the care required and suddenly finds themselves faced with nurses who have taken it over. Some nurses might still feel angry and say so but there are reasons why this may not be the most helpful reaction. To understand this, one has to consider the role of anxiety and unconscious defences against it. At some semi-conscious level, the relative may know that their accusations are unfair but if nurses become defensive and angry in response, this becomes a justification for the relative's anger to continue and possibly intensify. Nothing is understood, nothing resolved and it is likely that in future, nurses will try to avoid that relative as much as possible. Fighting is often preferable to facing the pain and guilt of helplessness and uselessness but if deeper feelings are faced, creative solutions may emerge. Both nurses and relatives may actually share intense anxiety in the face of their mutual helplessness, concerning the needs of some patients. Avoiding facing this may lead nurses to seek to be the all-important carer, thereby rendering relatives more useless than is necessary.

The 'blocking' that Macleod Clark (1981) drew attention to in her research needs to be understood, not as the ignorant responses of nurses who need to be educated to know better but as a semi-conscious, sometimes unconscious response to anxiety. Macleod Clark was familiar with the work of Menzies Lyth but she cannot square how it can be that nurses seemed to 'block' communication from patients, in situations that were not apparently stressful. Her suggestion is that 'the nurse was behaving in an automatic way simply from habit' (Macleod Clark, 1981). The solution to a bad habit is presumably some notion of breaking the habit, through example and training but this overlooks the possibility that such behaviour is an unconscious defence, a form of protection against too much anxiety and that the habitual 'blocking' of patient communication can be used as a total barrier, a permanent buffer against the possibility of distress arising in the nurse.

The anxiety of being flooded with emotional communications from patients that will distress and overwhelm nurses, leaving them feeling helpless and not knowing how to respond, is a reality of working closely with ill and dying people. The customary educative response helps in processing and containing such anxiety but it is insufficient to meet the full impact of the day-to-day work. What is needed is not instruction about what to do in such circumstances but better containment of the anxiety, in order to improve the nurse's capacity to contain the patient's anxiety. The containment of feeling can happen anywhere in skilful hands, so a classroom may be as good a place as any, but I would argue, it is more usually seen as a clinical rather than educative capacity because of its primary reliance on emotional attunement, rather than knowledge achieved through cognition. Symington (1990) refers to this distinction as 'emotional knowledge' and 'intellectual knowledge' and he says: 'In answer to the age-old question "Does knowledge liberate?", it seems clear that intellectual knowledge does not. It may free from ignorance but not from anxiety' (Symington, 1990, p. 99). Professional education seems to have difficulty in fully grasping the significance of this.

Ultimately, one wants some synthesis of emotional sensitivity, emotional strength, expressed through the capacity to tolerate strong feelings without being overwhelmed, and thought, which can give meaning to the processes at work. It is Bion (1959 and 1962, cited by Isaacs Elmhirst, 1981) who first used the word 'containment' in this way. He had in mind how a relaxed and competent mother (an emotional container) receives her baby's primitive and intense emotional expressions, thinks about them and responds in ways which modify the unbearable intensity for the baby. The feelings have to be first contained, that is, held in the mother's mind and reflected upon before action. Bion used the word 'reverie' for this activity. Any ensuing action aims to relieve the baby both physically and emotionally, so that the baby can start to grasp, over many repetitions, that the fearful and intolerable, can be less fearful and more tolerable. For the baby, this enables trust in the mother, the self and the world to accrue simultaneously. The reverse may happen if things go awry.

Thought used in isolation from the capacity to contain strong emotions, can be another way of simply trying to bypass the anxiety that is being expressed by patients. Reassurance would be one illustration of this. Reassurance involves telling someone who is worried that there is no need to worry and that their anxiety is therefore misplaced. This can work to diminish anxiety in circumstances where there is incorrect knowledge of the facts, which can then be put straight, but what people often get most anxious about is their fantasies about these facts. These fantasies, which may be conscious or unconscious are not straightforwardly amenable to dismissal by rational argument and factual clarification. I recall a man who was in an absolute panic as he watched the blood in his urine, during continuous irrigation following a trans-urethral resection of prostate. The nurses could tell him endlessly that this was normal and there was nothing to worry about. The reassurance did not touch him and the nurses became anxious, knowing that the patient's intense anxiety would increase his real chances of bleeding more, rather than less. They also felt irritated, as they did not know what to do, beyond suggesting sedation. What no-one did was to try to establish why the patient was in this panic, what it was that he thought/imagined was going on. To have been prepared to do this would have required a capacity to sit and listen, probably with a feeling of uselessness, alongside a person in some degree of terror and to wait until some understanding emerged. As Fabricius (1991, p.102) states, recalling the words of an experienced tutor, 'reassuring the patient was like isolating a fire with a fire blanket – it stopped you catching alight too and left the patient burning alone'.

An illustration of where time and space were given to understanding fantasy follows:

> An intern had as a patient a 42-year-old woman who was hospitalized with bronchial pneumonia. Although she was doing quite well, the intern asked her why she felt she had the illness. She was very relieved that he had asked her this question. She had recently undergone a hysterectomy and had become somewhat depressed after this surgery. She then developed the idea that there was an empty space in her body because of the hysterectomy. When she developed the pneumonia, she believed it was because this empty space had caused a draft in her bodily organs through her vagina. Although she was an intelligent woman, her life-long feelings of somehow being defective and inadequate were revived by the hysterectomy. Recognizing this, the intern was able to clarify the medical facts surrounding the hysterectomy and her pneumonia, and also to discuss some of her feelings that the hysterectomy had made her less of a woman (Blumenfield and Thomson 1985, p. 55).

One can see here how, given space and an interested listener, a person can speak clearly of their conscious fantasies about their illness and how a sensitive listener can also begin to get an idea of the unconscious ideas that may underpin these (hysterectomy as robbing her of her inside treasures and value as a woman perhaps). We all have *unconscious phantasies* (the 'ph' spelling is used to differentiate conscious fantasy from unconscious phantasy). They may serve to drive and shape the individual defence mechanisms that we use and also the social defences of groups of people working together, such as nurses (see Chapter 4).

Individual defence mechanisms

**Individual
defence
mechanisms**

One of these is *denial* which has already been mentioned. It is not possible here to go through the whole list of them, although these are easily found in books on psychology for nurses, for example McGhie (1979). A brief psychoanalytic overview is provided by Galatariotou (2005) and a rather complex account can also be found on Wikipedia.

http://en.wikipedia.org/wiki/Defence_mechanism.

This book will provide accounts of some common mechanisms, to include: *denial, regression, projection, projective identification* and *sublimation*. Brief attention will also be given to *displacement and manic defences*. This choice reflects the editors' belief that understanding these mechanisms in particular can be helpful to the task of nursing.

First, it is important to state what such mechanisms are, namely unconscious responses to protect us from too high levels of anxiety. We need them and it is not in our gift to select which ones we will use, although family patterns and genetic factors may influence this. Used rigidly and extensively, however, some defences may be counterproductive, as they interfere with our being able to face reality in life, for example, the person who uses denial to try and cope with loss is unable to adjust to it.

Projection is another frequently encountered mechanism. Our culture recognises this phenomenon in some proverbs, for example: 'It is a bad workman who blames his tools' and in some parables, for example, where one is exhorted not to comment on the splinter in one's brother's eye, lest one ignore the log in one's own (Luke 6:42). However, it was psychoanalysis that gave this a more theoretical and thus explanatory base. An example of projection is as follows: a teenage daughter of a friend of mine said, on failing her exams, that all her teachers were useless. One becomes suspicious with a remark like this because whilst some teachers might indeed be relatively useless, it is very unlikely that all were. Something, namely 'being useless' is being unfairly laid at their doorstep, in this instance, probably the teenager's own unbearable feeling of being useless by failing her exams. Projection involves trying to rid oneself of some unacceptable thought or feeling by locating it in someone else. The situation is frequently, however, more complicated than the previous example because we often choose to project into people who genuinely do exhibit something of the projected feeling, in their own right. For example, angry people are frequently angry but they can also become carriers of other people's unwanted angry feelings, through projection. This may make it hard for the angry individual to alter their position, as there is subtle, unconscious pressure from these other people to retain it. Projection is ubiquitous but in ordinary, well people, it may be a transient phenomenon which serves a purpose until one is able to cope better and reclaim the projections. Alternatively, people may settle comfortably into systems of mutual projection that suit everybody and work well. All marriages contain some degree of mutual projection which can be experienced as strengthening and supportive for the individuals within it. Nevertheless, some people get stuck in very rigid, projective patterns which restrict their ability to learn and be creative; the bully–victim system would be one such illustration.

The bully projects their own timidity and fear into someone else, usually someone perceived to be timid and weak in some way. The victim may also project their aggression, which they may be frightened of owning, into the bully who expresses it for them. In this system, the bully does not have to face their own weakness, timidity and fear and so is restricted emotionally from properly knowing who they are and of finding ways of coping with this, that are creative and not aggressive and destructive. The victim is similarly depleted by believing in their own weakness and not having their aggression available for appropriate use.

Nurses may project into patients unwell parts of themselves and patients may project into nurses well parts of themselves. If this system was very rigid, one would have to call it a 'sick' system, as nurses might be invested in patients not getting better, no matter what was said to the contrary! However, this plainly is not what ordinarily happens; nurses do help patients to get better. This system, therefore is not rigid but fluid and nurses may obtain a great deal of satisfaction in their work by identifying with the patient's recovery, so that they feel increasing confidence in their reparative capacities: this helps their internal situation (coping with unwell parts of the self) as well as the external situation (the ill patient recovers).

The nature of the unconscious

Difficulties occur in health care when nurses are overly burdened with very difficult projections from patients, for example being treated as if they were not good enough, when they are doing everything in their power to help, or being idealised when they feel themselves to be simply ordinary. The earlier quotation from Menzies Lyth (1988) made it clear just how difficult the world of health care can be. There is a further slant on projection called *projective identification* and this will be explored in Chapter 4.

Clinical supervision

Clinical supervision

What has been said so far leads to a plea in support of clinical supervision for nurses, a theme that will be explored further in Chapters 13 and 14. However, the capacity of any supervisor to contain the feelings of the supervisee and, thereby enhance that person's professional capacities, will only be as good as the supervisor's own experiences of containment. Containment for a supervisor means having the capacity to feel something of the feeling that the supervisee is trying to communicate and, like the mother described previously, being able to recognise it, accept it, name it and think about it, without panicking. This capacity will come from upbringing as well as professional experience and some people have a head-start over others. Ultimately, however, I would argue that there is a need to both teach and supervise supervisors, by persons experienced in identifying both conscious and unconscious aspects of interpersonal communication. The learning which occurs has to be experiential to allow for emotional growth which can be integrated with intellectual understanding.

Conclusion

This chapter has introduced and described a theory developed within psychoanalysis, notably by Sigmund Freud and his contemporaries, about the nature of the mind. This is to see it as comprising conscious, unconscious and pre-conscious components. These are to be understood as metaphors for capturing important distinctions in mental life, not as observable 'things' that could be seen under a microscope, as one might investigate areas of the brain. Examples have been given to show how ubiquitous unconscious phenomena are, with 'slips of the tongue', 'forgetting' and the emotional defence of 'denial' in bereavement. The relevance of this for nursing has been demonstrated with reference to understanding some nurse–patient interactions with a particular focus on defence mechanisms; denial and projection have been examined. The significance of clinical supervision is acknowledged and will be a recurrent theme pursued throughout this book. All the chapters which now follow will expand upon this idea of the relevance of 'the unconscious' to nursing theory and practice.

References

Bion, W.R. (1959). *Experiences in Groups*. London: Tavistock.

Bion, W.R. (1962). *Learning from Experience*, London: Paul Heinnemann.

Blumenfield, M and Thokpson, T. (1985). The psychological reactions to physical illness. In *Understanding Human Behaviour in Health and Illness*, ed. R. Simons, 3rd edn. London: Williams and Wilkins pp.48–59.

Fabricius, J. (1991). 'Running on the spot or can nursing really change?' *Psychoanalytic Psychotherapy* 5 (2): 97–108.

Fairbairn, G. and Mead, D. (1990). 'Ethics and the loss of innocence.' *Paediatric Nursing* 2 (5): 22–23.

Freud, S. (2001). 'The ego and the id' [1923]. In *The Standard Edition of the Complete Psychological Works of Sigmund Freud*, vol. XIX. London: Vintage (The Hogarth Press) pp.12–66.

Galatariotou, C. (2005). 'The defences.' In *Introducing Psychoanalysis: Essential Themes and Topic*, eds. S. Budd and R. Rusbridger. London: Routledge, pp. 15–38.

Isaacs Elmhirst, S. (1981). 'Bion and babies.' In *Do I Dare Disturb the Universe? A Memorial to Wilfred R.Bion*. Beverley Hills, California: Caesura Press, pp.84–91.

Kandel, E. (1999). 'Biology and the future of psychoanalysis: a new intellectual framework for psychiatry revisited.' *American Journal of Psychiatry* 156, April: 505–24.

Laplanche, J. and Pontalis, J.-B. (1988). *The Language of Psychoanalysis*. London: Karnac Books.

Luke 6:42, *The New Jerusalem Bible*.

Macleod Clark, J. (1981). 'Communications in nursing.' Nursing Times 77, Jan. 1, pp. 12–18.

McGhie, A. (1979). *Psychology as Applied to Nursing*. 7th edn. London: Churchill

Livingstone.

Menzies Lyth, I. (1988). *Containing Anxiety in Institutions*, Vol 1. London: Free Association Books.

Mollon, P. (2000). *The Unconscious. Ideas in Psychoanalysis Series.* Duxford, Cambridge: Icon Books Ltd.

Ryle, G. (1963). *The Concept of Mind.* Harmondsworth, Middx.: Penguin.

Schore, A.. (1993). *Affect Regulation and the Origin of the Self.* New York: Jason Aronson.

Shaffer, P. (2006). *Equus.* London: Penguin Books Ltd.

Stockwell, F. (1972). *The Unpopular Patient.* London: Royal College of Nursing.

Symington, N. (1990). 'The possibility of human freedom and its transmission (with particular reference to the thought of Bion).' *International Journal of Psychoanalysis* 71: 95–106.

Wikipedia http://en.wikipedia.org/wiki/Defence_mechanism (Accessed 13 July 2008)

Chapter 2
Developing relationships
Mary Paget

Introduction

Most nurses seem to intuitively understand the patient's concerns, but there are times when their relationships with their patients become fraught, tense or difficult. Although it is often easy to attribute this to the patient's feelings of concern, anxiety and fear, there are also times when nurses find it difficult to understand why these tensions exist. In this chapter, the theories of attachment and object relations will be considered in an attempt to illuminate the ways in which an infant's first relationships with key caregivers can influence subsequent relationships throughout life. Frequent reference will be made to 'mother'. This encompasses the range of people that could be held to be the main care-giver of the infant, so will include the natural mother, the father, foster parent, etc.

Most people are familiar with the suggestion that all human beings make bonds with others. Such emotional connections with a number of individuals serve a range of purposes, from family relationships to friendships and working relationships; even transient relationships can give rise to an emotional connection. These relationships incur some level of responsibility, for example, in a working relationship there is often the need to give mutual support. Within most families, such relationships and responsibilities are much more complex, with roles of giving, taking, supporting and caring in accordance with needs.

An affectional bond is a form of attachment, where one individual has great emotional significance for another (Ainsworth, 2005). Any individual has a number of affectional bonds, each different. Thus, they are never entirely interchangeable with or replaceable by another affectional bond. This ability to interact with others emotionally is important throughout life, providing comfort, security, companionship and support.

Bowlby (2005) suggests that such bonds or attachments also serve more significant purposes; he considers that bonds of attachment are fundamental to the development of all children and retain significance throughout adulthood and old age. Indeed, Bowlby (2005) considers that attachments made in infancy are necessary for the survival of that infant and act as a foundation for all the other attachments made throughout life. Freud (1856–1939) coined the phrase that the 'child is father to the man' and suggested that a loving relationship with the mother is indispensable to the growing infant (cited in Bowlby, 2005, p. 7).

Attachment theory has been developed from Bowlby's original work and attempts to explain the ways in which the relationship between mother and baby directly affects the psychological coping strategies of the developing child. Winnicott (1988) suggests such facilitation of early emotional development by the mother helps the baby to develop strategies with which to face a difficult world. Such strategies are carried on into adolescence, with early attachment experiences providing a basis for entering into peer relationships. As development continues, early attachment strategies and family and peer experiences form the foundations for more mature intimate relationships. In this way, attachment theory can be used to interpret relationships and resulting psychological difficulties in adulthood.

At this point, it is appropriate to question the validity of such a theory and ask what evidence exists to support its main tenets. Bowlby adopted a careful, questioning approach to theorising, using observational studies conducted by Robertson and Robertson (for example, *A two-year-old goes to hospital*, film, 1953), reviewing data from studies of infants' cognitive and social development and Ainsworth's (1967) study of children in Uganda. Bowlby's early theory and scientific approach have stimulated debate and a considerable body of research, with a number of longitudinal studies of children observed during infancy and in later years (Grossman, Grossman and Waters 2005). Consequently, there is a growing body of clinical evidence to support the utility of these theories.

Attachment and personal development

Attachment and personal development

Prior to Bowlby's (1991) publication of his early views on attachment behaviour, several key assumptions existed about the nature and origins of a child's tie with its mother, based on a number of instinctive responses (Bowlby, 1991, p. 178). The first is that the child has a range of physiological needs, particularly for food and warmth, which the mother meets. In due course, the baby learns that she is the source of gratification and becomes interested in and attached to her.

The second premise suggests that infants have an instinctive propensity to attach themselves to the human breast, or substitute and to suck it and to 'possess it orally'. The infant learns that attached to this breast is a mother and, with time, comes to relate to her. Finally, infants need to touch and cling to another human being; this is independent of the need for food and warmth, but is satisfied during feeding and holding.

Bowlby (1991) postulated that a child's tie to its mother is a product of the behavioural premises described. From the very beginning, the child's many needs make it essential that the mother makes a very close adaptation to the child. The mother learns when the child needs to be turned, fed, cuddled and how to manage the child when it is upset. These activities by their nature, result in the mother's proximity to the child and through this, attachment is established. The child learns to maintain this proximity by using strategies such as smiling, which draws the mother to the child, or by using more aversive behaviours, such as crying which have the same effect (Fonagy, 2001). On achieving independent mobility, the child will use this ability to stay close to the mother, who represents safety and security.

The sense of safety and security fostered by the proximity to the mother allows the child to play contentedly and to explore its environment. Ainsworth (1967) described this as an 'exploratory behaviour system', with the attachment figure providing an essential 'secure base' from which to explore. However, anything threatening the infant's perception of its own safety or security, such as the absence of the mother or the presence of a stranger provokes a range of typical attachment behaviours, described by Bowlby (1991) as the 'fear system'. The typical behaviour is a tendency to regain and maintain proximity to the mother. With threat, the distance between mother and child is reduced, with the infant typically seeking mother's arms. Any threat to the continued presence of the mother provokes strong protest and active attempts to prevent the separation. Bowlby coined the phrase 'separation protest' to describe this behaviour. Typically, the child becomes acutely distressed and uses all available strategies to regain the mother: crying, calling and looking eagerly towards any sight or sound that may indicate mother's return, but rejecting any offers of comfort from alternative figures. Should mother not return, as seen in *A two-year-old goes to Hospital* (1953) (which showed what occurred when a small child was separated from mother through hospitalisation) the child becomes increasingly withdrawn and inactive, generally detached from normal play, but accepting care from alternative figures (Robertson, 1952). Comparisons can be made with the behaviour of bereaved persons. In adulthood, the dawning recognition of a permanent loss is accompanied by calling, crying and searching for the lost one, a feeling of restlessness and despair and a persistent perceptual recall of the loved one; the constant 'listening for the latch'.

Additionally, Bowlby (1991) describes a situation where, following a period of separation, the child may refuse to greet its mother, instead appearing to reject her and remaining indifferent to her advances. Together, the attachment behaviours, the exploratory behavioural system, the fear system and the responses of the mother-figure are thought to influence the way that the child copes with stressors and adapts its behaviours during psychological development. An example of this would be the way in which a secure child learns to cope with mother's brief absences with increasing confidence.

The secure base

This aspect of attachment theory was initially developed by Blatz (1940) and further developed by Bowlby and Ainsworth in the context of attachment. As suggested earlier, one important aspect of the behaviour of small children is the need to maintain proximity to mother, as a source of familiarity and security. This security forms a base from which the child can gradually work outwards, developing new skills and interests away from mother. In a strange situation, such as the first day in a playgroup, the small child will be unsure of its surroundings, but, with mother within view, will sooner or later begin to explore. This exploratory activity is important, as it contributes to the child's developing levels of self reliance and their coping strategies. The child will return to be close to mother at the first suggestion of threat; a loud noise, a new face or even a new object may be perceived as threatening and stimulate this return to mother's arms for comfort, reassurance and security.

Conversely, when at home in a familiar environment, the child is less likely to feel insecure, even when mother leaves the room and is out of sight. In these circumstances, the child is likely to simply search for its mother, or call out for her attention. Only if the absence is prolonged will the child resort to crying. Security therefore, can be engendered either through the support of a figure of attachment or through familiarity of environment, which is associated with the attachment figure. Main (2005) suggests that when the child is confident of the caregiver's support, the security of this knowledge frees the child from the burden of constantly monitoring their caregiver's physical whereabouts and psychological availability. However, the absence of the mother in a strange situation can trigger feelings of insecurity and distress (Ainsworth *et al.*, 1978).

Sroufe and Waters (1977) linked this to a sense of 'felt security', considering that there is more to the phenomenon than just the regulation of physical distance. The internal world of the child, its mood or whether or not it is feeling unwell may also influence the child's sense of security at any given time. How a child responds to separation, the social environment or external events will reflect their sense of 'felt security'. The provision of a secure base needs to be properly emphasised, as it remains necessary throughout a child's development (Sroufe *et al.*, 2005). Bowlby (2005) adds that the secure base has clear value in early years and is no less important during adolescence and more mature years. He considers that people of all ages are best able to develop and deploy their talents when they have a trusted person to give aid or support, although this may be less obvious in mature adults. This trusted figure provides a 'secure base' from which to operate.

Ainsworth *et al.* (1978) devised a simple laboratory experiment, now known as the 'Strange Situation', in order to observe attachment behaviours in small children under two years of age. In this experiment, she monitored the behaviour of children during two brief (thirty second to three minute) periods of separation from their mothers. In the first episode, the mother simply leaves the room for a very short period of time; in the second, a stranger enters the room. Each child's behaviour during the stressful time of separation and also during reunion was then compared with its usual behaviour in the home environment. From this research, four distinctive styles of attachment behaviour emerged, which can be strongly linked to the nature of the child's relationship with its mother in the home situation.

Securely attached children play and explore happily prior to separation and openly demonstrate immediate distress on separation, but are easily comforted on reunion. Such infants have parents who help them manage emotions in a balanced and controlled way and their behaviour reflects an internal confidence that the mother will return and will help them manage their distressed feelings (Steele and Steele, 2005).

The *anxiously attached, avoidant* type of behaviour is demonstrated when the child is seen to be trying to suppress emotions at separation and affect an attitude of disinterest upon reunion. When the mother returns, the infant ignores and avoids her, focusing its attention on its toys or moving away from the mother. When observed in the home environment, the mother is seen to be particularly unresponsive to overt evidence of the child's distress. Such infants have learned that it is better to pretend that all is well, even when deep inside, they are experiencing distress. This is thought to indicate a lack of confidence in the mother's availability. This behaviour is also seen in later years, for example, the aged patient in hospital who appears to 'punish' their family members by ignoring them when they come to visit.

The *anxiously ambivalent/resistant* child shows distress at separation but is not comforted by the mother's return. The child seems to exaggerate its responses in order to ensure its mother's attention, sometimes kicking at or smacking the mother. The child has learned to overtly display intense negative emotions, with no clear expectation that its needs will be met. Haft and Slade (1989) consider that such children are likely to have been cared for by parents who ignore or misconstrue their emotional signals. Parallels can be drawn with aged patients who constantly call for attention and are often petulant.

Finally, the *disorganised/disoriented* child is likely to remain distressed long after its separation from its mother is over. The child continues to seek proximity to its mother, but displays contradictory behaviour, for example by approaching its mother cautiously, or even by hiding close by. Main and Hesse (1990) linked this form of attachment to frightened or frightening caregiving, suggesting that infants cannot reconcile the paradox of fearing the figures they yearn to approach for comfort in times of distress. Carlsson *et al.* (1989) suggest that children who are abused may demonstrate this form of extreme disorganisation while still manifesting attachment to their abuser. Aged people who are abused may demonstrate similar behaviour.

Longitudinal studies (Crowell and Waters, 2005, Main, Hesse and Kaplan, 2005, both cited in Grossman, Grossman and Waters, 2005) suggest that the presence or absence of attachment figures affects the development of personality functioning and the ability to initiate and to maintain mutually rewarding relationships. As adults, secure individuals are more likely to have developed a positive image of themselves (Nathanson, 1987). A healthy adult person is one who is able to act as a secure base for others when necessary. At other times, this person will rely on others for a secure base. Inconsistent or absent attachment figures lead to impaired functioning, typified by an inability to collaborate in rewarding relationships, with anxious clinging and excessive demands, or non-committal relationships and defiant independence (Bowlby, 2005). In Salter's words (1940) the person has been 'handicapped by... the lack of a secure base' (Salter, 1940, p. 45).

Attachment theory and object relations

Attachment theory

Both object relations and attachment theory developed from psychoanalytic thinking but until recently were different branches of thought with little dialogue between them. Attachment theorists have tended to see attachment as a consequence of the satisfaction of instinctual drives. In contrast, object relations theory places relationships at the heart of a person's psychological development. The 'object' referred to is not an inanimate object, rather it refers to the desire to initiate and maintain relationships with others. Gomez (1998) considers that the need for a relationship with a key person (usually the mother) is the primary driving force and that instincts and drives are subordinated to this need. Enduring relationships have both survival value and provide a sense of satisfaction, but the way that relationships are sustained often reflects the environment in which early relationships are developed. Ainsworth's Strange Situation, in particular, demonstrates the ways in which the behaviour of small children upon reunion, mirrors the internalised strategies they have learned from the specific caregiver they are observed with.

Clinicians are familiar with the notion that certain behaviours (such as abuse) can be learned in childhood and replicated later when that child is itself a parent, thus perpetuating a cycle of abuse that passes from generation to generation. Similarly 'good parenting' is learned as a child and can also be passed down through generations. Given this fact, a number of writers (Bowlby, 2005, Ainsworth, 2005) have commented on the importance of nurturing attachment relationships appropriately, linking poor attachment experiences with long-term mental health problems, the inability to develop coping strategies and to form and maintain affectional bonds.

Object relations

Object relations

As a result of working as a psychoanalyst with a range of children and adults, Melanie Klein (1959) considered that many of their problems had links to the earliest infantile feelings about their parents and siblings, opening up the idea that each of us has an inner world, which interacts with and influences our perceptions of the external world. She theorised that even the smallest infant has a complex and unconscious 'internal world' populated by its impressions of those people closest to it, combined with a range of anxieties about its experience of the world. The infant's inner world is filled with phantasies (spelled with a 'ph' to distinguish unconscious phantasies from conscious fantasies), and figures within this internal world are experienced as if they concretely exist. Monsters are real for the small infant. It is surmised that the baby lives in a world where inner and outer experiences are undifferentiated and with no demarcation between dreaming and reality. As the infant develops through to childhood and adulthood, the capacity to make this distinction increases. The internal world becomes increasingly complex, formed as it is by our earliest relationships, our experiences, feelings, anxieties and phantasies. This internal world is like a filter, through which we perceive and comprehend the external world. Klein (1959) identified two key states of mind, present in early infant development but continuing throughout life. She referred to these as the paranoid-schizoid position and the depressive position. The former precedes the latter.

The paranoid-schizoid position

To understand the paranoid-schizoid position, one must first consider the newborn infant. It has no sense of time, has no language with which to think or to communicate and its main sensations will relate to being fed, held, bathed or talked to. It has no idea of the boundaries of its own body, so cannot differentiate between itself and others. This un-integrated emotional state is thought to give rise to many conflicts leading to persecutory anxieties, or terrors.

Klein (1959) coined the phrase 'the good breast' to refer to those elements that give the infant comfort: food from the nurturing breast, arms that cradle it or the voice that soothes it. The 'good breast' becomes a good 'internal object' which relieves the baby's anxieties. As the baby cannot differentiate between himself and the 'good breast', he initially believes that he is himself the source of the good feelings. Similarly, uncomfortable feelings of hunger, frustration and anger cause feelings of distress and anxiety which are difficult for the infant to cope with. To cope with these feelings, the infant learns to attribute the bad feelings to a persecutory object, a process of 'splitting' these feelings away from his representation of himself and attributing them to something else: the 'bad breast'. This process of disowning persecutory feelings and attributing them to something or someone else forms the basis of the notion of projective identification. Essentially a primitive mechanism, it can resurface in adults at times of stress (see Chapter 4 for further discussion of projective identification).

According to Bion (1959) the role of the mother is to act as a receiver or container for her child's emotions and to accept, absorb and transform these overwhelming and persecutory feelings into some form of meaning. This allows the infant to cope with and re-internalise these feelings in a way that is tolerable. This process continues until such a time that the infant learns to do this for himself, but if it does not occur effectively, then defensive structures are thought to develop in the infant, which in turn can influence and impede its emotional development. Unlike attachment theorists, object relations theorists do not talk of managing or controlling emotions but rather of 'containing' them. The idea is that through being emotionally contained by our parents in our childhood, we become reasonably self-contained as adults. Vocabulary such as 'controlling' or 'managing' feelings is eschewed because it tends to suggest defensive manoeuvres such as 'minimisation' or 'denial', which are the antithesis of containment. Containment allows the individual to recognise and analyse their emotions, facilitating their recognition as a foundation for further development and growth.

The depressive position

As the child grows, from the age of about three months, it develops the capacity to see the mother as a whole and separate object, accounting for both good and bad experiences. According to Klein (1959), this is accompanied by the infant's own awareness of its capacity to both love and hate the mother. This ambivalence opens up feelings of guilt in the infant and is termed the 'depressive position'. As the need to split off bad feelings diminishes, experiences are perceived differently. As Gomez phrases it 'the bad is less bad, but by the same token, the good is less good' (1998, p. 42). The infant becomes aware that the mother it hates when in a rage is the same mother it loves when times are good between them. This painful recognition slowly enables the child to become more tolerant of its own mixed emotions, with less necessity to eject and project them into others.

It is important to recognise that the depressive position is not the same as a clinical state of depression. In the depressive position, the guilt felt is of a remorseful rather than persecutory nature, paving the way for efforts at reparation, a sense that although anger can damage, love can mend. Gomez (1998) gives a good example of this:

We see young children repeatedly working through experiences of persecution, loss, guilt and reparation; tantrums and conflict alternate with an absolute need for love and an urgent necessity to give. Many are the cold cups of 'tea' which parents have been roused with at 5 a.m., and the grubby bits of biscuit offered for their enjoyment. Parents know, without necessarily knowing why, that to reject these gifts would be a crushing blow to their child's sense of having something good to give. These early forms of reparation develop into helpfulness and individual interests and talents, all ways of contributing to society. (Gomez, 1998, p. 43)

It was Klein's contention that whilst the depressive position is first encountered and hopefully negotiated in infancy, the need to move from the paranoid-schizoid position to the depressive position is a constant requirement to successfully respond to life's challenges. At different times, we feel either more or less confident, more or less secure. We face up to or hide from issues of concern, depending on our ability to see things with different degrees of clarity. Human creativity stems from the repeated, successful negotiation of the depressive position, but those who get stuck in the paranoid-schizoid position may not be able to live lives that make the most of their inherent potential. Chapter 4 gives an illustration of a group of nurses and doctors moving from the paranoid-schizoid position to the depressive position, with beneficial consequences for the care of their patients.

Conclusion

Many theorists believe that attachments of childhood influence the attachment relationships of adulthood. Although the nature of the relationships may change, the need for such relationships does not diminish throughout life. Both attachment theory and object relations theory offer a flexible framework that can assist nurses to understand the nature of relationships and the ways in which relationships can affect behaviour. For an effective nurse/patient relationship to develop, nurses must pay attention to their own emotions as well as those of their patients, being careful to consider their patients' feelings and attitudes, as well as their own hunches. This may allow nurses to work with and to understand other people, particularly those whose behaviour appears baffling or unpredictable.

References

A Two-Year-Old Goes to Hospital (Film, 1953). Made by J. Robertson and J.A. Robertson. London: Tavistock Child Development Research Unit.

Ainsworth, M. (1967). *Infancy in Uganda*. Baltimore: Johns Hopkins.

Ainsworth, M. (2005). 'Attachments and other affectional bonds' [1991]. In *Attachment Across the Life Cycle,* eds. C. Murray Parkes, J. Stevenson-Hinde and P. Marris. London: Routledge, pp. 33–51.

Ainsworth, M., Blehar, M.C., Waters, E. and Wall, S. (1978). *Patterns of Attachment: A Psychological Study of the Strange Situation*. Hillsdale NJ: Erlbaum.

Bion, W.R. (1959). 'Attacks on linking.' *International Journal of Psychoanalysis* 40: 308–15.

Blatz, W. (1940). *Hostages to Peace: Parents and the Children of Democracy*. New York: Morrow.

Bowlby, J. (1991). *Attachment and Loss: Volume 1. (Attachment)*. London: Penguin.

Bowlby, J. (2005). *The Making and Breaking of Affectional Bonds*. London: Routledge Classics.

Carlsson, V., Cicchetti, D., Barnett, D. and Braunwald, K. (1989). 'Disorganised/disoriented attachment relationships in maltreated infants.' *Developmental Psychology* 25: 525–31.

Crowell, J. and Waters, E. (2005). 'Attachment representations, secure-base behaviour and the evolution of adult relationships: the Stony Brook adult relationship project.' In *Attachment from Infancy to Adulthood: the Major Longitudinal Studies*, eds. K.E. Grossman, K. Grossman and E. Waters. New York: The Guilford Press, pp.223–44.

Fonagy, P. (2001). *Attachment Theory and Psychoanalysis*. New York: Other Press.

Gomez, L. (1998). *An Introduction to Object Relations*. London: Free Association Books.

Grossman, K.E., Grossman, K. and Waters, E. (eds) (2005). *Attachment from Infancy to Adulthood: the Major Longitudinal Studies*, New York: The Guilford Press.

Haft, W. and Slade, A. (1989). 'Affect attunement and maternal attachment: a pilot study.' *Infant Mental Health Journal* 10: 157–72.

Klein, M. (1959). 'Our adult world and its roots in infancy.' *Human Relations* 12: 291–303.

Main, M. (2005). 'Metacognitive knowledge, metacognitive monitoring and singular (coherent) vs. multiple (incoherent) model of attachment: findings and direction for future research' [1991]. In *Attachment Across the Life Cycle*, eds. C. Murray Parkes, J. Stevenson- Hinde and P. Marris. London: Routledge, pp.127–59.

Main, M. and Hesse, E. (1990). 'Parents' unresolved traumatic experiences are related to infant disorganised attachment status: is frightened and/or frightening parental behaviour the linking mechanism?' In *Attachment in the Preschool Years: Theory, Research and Intervention*, eds M. Greenberg, D. Cicchetti and E.M. Cummings. Chicago: University of Chicago Press, pp. 161–82.

Main, M., Hesse, E. and Kaplan, N. (2005). 'Predictability of attachment behaviour and representational processes at 1, 6 and 19 years of age: the Berkeley longitudinal study.' In *Attachment from Infancy to Adulthood: the Major Longitudinal Studies*, eds. K.E. Grossman, K. Grossman and E. Waters. New York: The Guilford Press, pp. 245–304.

Nathanson, D.L. (1987). *The Many Faces of Shame*. New York: The Guilford Press.

Robertson, J. (1952). *A two-year-old goes to hospital* (Film). London: Tavistock Child Development Research Unit.

Robertson, J. A., (1953). 'Some responses of young children to loss of maternal care.' *Nursing Care* **49**: 382–86.

Salter, M.D. (1940). *An Evaluation of Adjustment Based upon the Concept of Security. Child Development Series*. Toronto: The University of Toronto Press.

Sroufe, L.A. and Waters, E. (1977). 'Attachment as an organisational construct.' *Child Development* **48**: 1184–99.

Sroufe, L.A., Egeland, B., Carlson, E. and Collins, W.A. (2005). 'Placing early attachment experiences in developmental context.' In *Attachment from Infancy to Adulthood: the Major Longitudinal Studies*, eds. K.E. Grossman, K. Grossman and E. Waters. New York: The Guilford Press, pp. 48–70.

Steele, H. and Steele, M. (2005). 'Understanding and resolving emotional conflict. The London parent-child project.' In *Attachment from Infancy to Adulthood: the Major Longitudinal Studies*, eds. K.E. Grossman, K. Grossman and E. Waters. New York: The Guilford Press, pp.137–64.

Winnicott, D.W. (1988). *Babies and Their Mothers*. London: Free Association Books.

Chapter 3
The experience of illness and loss
Mic Rafferty

Introduction

The intent of the chapter is to reveal and illuminate the human condition of illness, as a change experience involving loss. Attention is focused on the emotional and interpersonal nature of illness, informed by psychodynamic understandings, primarily to enable empathic understanding. Furthermore, such information can inform practice, as understanding the dynamic nature of loss reactions helps to establish how as nurses, we can best enable another. The empathic act is to have an emotional understanding of another's experience, informed by knowledge. For nursing practice, the influence of knowledge is perhaps the most important aspect of empathy. It makes it possible to know 'a truth about significant life issues' (Black, 2001) giving a shape of meaning to 'the intensely personal, highly emotional often brutal predicaments lived by patients', which informs us about what we can do, this 'makes the difference' (Koch, 1998, p.1183).

There is no better illustration of the impact of psychodynamic insights informing the empathic interpretation of experience, than the profound transformation in understanding that resulted from the pioneering work of the Robertsons (1971) leading to major changes in the nursing care of hospitalised children and their families. They showed that children separated from their mothers because of hospitalisation were not quietly accepting, but rather profoundly depressed. Indeed, if today one shows to student nurses one of the Robertsons' films, charting a child's response to parental separation, one is likely to meet accusations that it was a consciously cruel experiment.

Work undertaken by psychoanalysts has had an impact in understanding the human responses to loss, be that the loss of a spouse, a limb, a home, a community and indeed the final loss, which is death. Such understanding provides frames of reference to make better, but never complete sense of the complex 'maze of emotion and sensation' that is profound and sudden loss, in order to arrive at an appreciation of the experience (Murray Parkes 1988). The intention is to explain and illustrate such psychodynamic explanations of responses to threat and loss, by giving attention to what happens when we are ill, including how we defend ourselves and manage those threats and life transitions that illness may precipitate. Use will be made of qualitative research studies, which interpret concepts such as suffering, into the subjective meaning for the sufferer (Black, 2001, p. 294), providing insights into human experiences, which inform rather more than any medical formulation of a condition could do.

All who read this chapter have insights into the loss of a loved other, probably at a personal level. This much-studied reality has led to formulations of its character, giving psychological understanding of an often-wretched experience. For instance Murray Parkes (1971, p. 103.) who identifies the 'psychosocial transitional responses to the loss of a loved one', suggests the initial reaction is *numbness*, characterised by retreat into self-absorption, feelings of deadness, disbelief and sometimes denial, interrupted by outbursts of extremely intense distress or anger. *Yearning* and *searching* for the Dead follows, along with the social requirement to bury the Dead and mourn with others. Any eulogy, while primarily a celebration of a life is also about *yearning*, which fills a mind and body with memories and feelings in an attempt to bring the person back. *Searching* can range from the euphoria, followed by wretchedness that occurs when 'again hearing the door latch at four', to finding another eventually 'just like the dead one'. The phase of *disorgani-sation* and *despair* pays testament to the mental chaos caused by gaps left by the dead, when facing the grim task of enduring and surviving. The phase of greater or lesser degrees of *reorganisation* gives recognition to that time of grieving which is about claiming back an existence from the dead, while recognising that for many, the haunting loss never heals. There are many human versions of the grief experience and it is important to recognise that the loss of another can lead to outcomes that are about the flowering of human potential, when in some way freed from a co-existence with the dead person. That there can eventually be a 'bright side' to loss is exemplified by the many individuals and groups who have used the tragic loss of loved ones, to begin a quest for justice, reform, forgiveness or reconciliation. This capacity to sublimate, the unconscious diversion of energy from absorption with the dead person to creative acts that can benefit others, is perhaps the most inspiring quality of humanity.

This illustration in many ways sums up the experience of loss of whatever kind. Any major loss needs to be understood as shattering a life of meaning, which we do not give up without fight or protest, and which eventually leads to a transformation of the meaning of life, tied in a helpful or unhelpful way to what has been lost. Therefore, an understanding of the dynamics of this conservative impulse to resist change and loss (Marris 1986) is an important part of nursing knowledge, particularly when applied to illness.

The nature of loss and illness

The loss of a world of assumptions

The nature of loss and illness

To begin to appreciate the challenge presented by illness, it is worth recognising that 'the body is the embodiment of who we are' (Corbin, 2003, p. 256), with 'self' becoming what it is through the body and that in health 'the body is passed over in silence' (van Manen, 1998, p.11) and generally taken for granted. Sparkes (1998, pp.651–60) vividly captures the collapse of a world of body assumptions in a narrative study of an athlete, dealing with the loss of 'a high-performance body', accompanied by 'feelings of loss and fragmentation'. To describe this, Sparkes uses Athens (1995) who identifies a breaking apart of the old self via a traumatising social experience. This is so utterly foreign to the person that they cannot assimilate it, as it shatters taken-for-granted assumptions about their body, throwing them into a state of utter shock, disbelief and, finally, total disarray. Sparkes (1998) charts over time what it is for this individual to experience 'the demise of the disciplined body-self', loss of the 'gloried self', accompanied by the need to 'hold on to past selves'. We try desperately to hold on to our past selves, because without this we are helpless and lost (Marris, 1986).

Illness means some degree of assault upon, or indeed the collapse of the sufferer's sense of meaningful existence. Why this is the case lies in understanding the significance of early life experience 'in setting in stone the way things should be' (Holroyd, 2003, p. 6), so establishing a cumulative notion of what it is to be human. This is based on what we learn to expect, as the ordered and predictable state of affairs concerning love, family, community and the life cycle, leading to beliefs about ourselves as individuals, our physical bodies and our contribution to human affairs. Thus, loss and illness have the potential to challenge our system for predicting future events, as they threaten our basic assumptions and potentially our emotional attachments (Marris, 1986, p. 9). This provokes a deep-seated impulse to defend what we have learned to accept, for without such understanding, we risk becoming powerless and directionless.

The childhood roots of our assumptive world lie in primitive wants and the ways parental figures met or did not meet such wants, so establishing preverbal patterns and associations with pleasure or distress. If all goes well, such patterns give the child the notion they are secure and able to deal with their wants and needs because of reliable others, so establishing the thread of continuity and, thereby, freeing the inherent capacity to explore and change (see Chapter 2). It is important to remember that our ability to learn from experience, to change, relies on our capacity to place new experiences within a familiar, reliable construction of reality, originating from emotional attachments (Marris, 1986, pp. 6–7). The important part emotional attachments play in the consolidation of reality (Bowlby and Murray Parkes, 1970) enables an understanding of why it is so difficult to change social understandings, as this requires something more than just knowledge. The power of early emotional scripting upon attitudes to health and illness is demonstrated by Lubkin and Larsen's (2002, p. 24) work on illness behaviour. They suggest past experiences (for instance, observing one's parents being stoic, working when ill, avoiding medical help) influence children's future responses, as they assimilate them and mirror them in their own lives. As Black (2001, p. 294) observes: 'an already-fashioned self comes to the illness or dying experience with an identity shaped and woven through a personal and communal history' that begins within the family and is influenced by family and social scripts about what is gender, race, class, and age-appropriate behaviour.

The experience of illness and loss

Common reactions to illness

The body speaks to us through sensations anchored in meaning (Corbin, 2003) about what it is to be well or perhaps more accurately, to be ourselves. With illness, the familiar body becomes the unfamiliar body (Corbin, 2003), with the need to anchor unfamiliar sensations in meaning (Baker, 1998). Whatever the nature or seriousness of an illness, 'what if?' and 'what to do?' reactions are prompted, drawn from our assumptive worldview. Such 'what if?' and 'what to do?' reactions are conscious and unconscious defence mechanisms, protective in nature, as they relieve anxiety and guilt arising from fears, feelings, wishes, and thoughts (Blumenfield and Thompson, 1985). In understanding unconscious mental defences, it is important to realise they are ego defences against intolerable anxiety and ways of dealing instinctively, without thought, to threat (see also Chapters 1 and 4).

Bowlby (1969) suggests the best way to describe our assumptive world is as 'our world model', which includes ideal and dreaded derivates of the nature of our world. Anticipation of such 'might be worlds', for instance in day dreams about winning the lottery, or worries about losing a child, provide opportunities to rehearse, emotionally and mentally, such futures. Inevitably, the real thing throws up unexpected gaps and deficits in our ability to cope, provoking anxiety (Chapter 5 illustrates this). With regard to illness, this idea may help us to understand how such gaps and deficits, and the resulting anxiety, may engage the emotional defences of *minimisation*, *denial*, and *regression*.

Minimisation of illness is initially an adaptive response. Explaining away unfamiliar body sensations, such as breathlessness, pain, lethargy, as unimportant, is normally because of the counterweight of some social assumption, which must not be neglected. For example, concerning gender, a mother's priority may be to put her family's needs first, with unusual body sensations, a forgettable second. Skew (2005), a former president of the British Institute of Musculoskeletal Medicine, states that mothers typically report back pain when their youngest child is a teenager, with the original injury often occurring within a year of the last pregnancy. Skew claims 'Mothers don't have time to worry about minor aches and pains'(Skew 2005). Similarly, for many men, work identity is so important that 'giving in' to illness is unacceptable. Kivimäki *et al.* (2005) identify this phenomenon as 'sickness presenteeism' in a study about unhealthy male civil servants, which showed those who took no absence in a three-year period had twice as high an incidence of serious coronary events, than unhealthy employees with moderate levels of sickness absenteeism. Men are reportedly (Channel 4, 2008) notoriously reluctant to visit the doctor, often refusing to accept the seriousness of their condition and only seeking medical advice when there is obviously something wrong. Even then, they may delay, through a combination of denial and fatalism. It is important to recognise that socio-economic position, which inevitably mirrors class, racial, and gender realities, means that many at the bottom of the economic ladder cannot afford to 'throw a sickie', preferring to minimise illness and distress, until it seriously impacts upon their usual abilities and activities. *Minimisation* begins to border on *denial* when, for example, elderly people minimise health issues requiring attention, by dismissing them as something expected with age. Howse *et al.* (2005) suggest that elderly people can express denial in various ways, such as rejecting a diagnosis ('I do not have cancer'), minimising its implications ('yes I have cancer, but I'll live a good many years yet') or by appearing indifferent to it.

Denial is most graspable through illustrations evoking stark and dramatic predicaments, such as the initial emotional reaction following the death of a loved one, or a diagnosis of terminal cancer, when the person is not able to accept their loss or diagnosis. This initial denial protects from the emotional shock and intense grief that often accompanies loss. It is important to keep in mind that denial is a response to an unbearable threat. This threat to our assumptive world has to be psychically pushed away, making it possible to see that denial may take many forms, including illusory positivism, disregard and anger.

The account of a disabled person (Ouch's blog, 2008) captures well the pitfalls of illusory positivism:

I spent an *age* in denial about my illness. My prognosis was always uncertain, so I assumed that it was a matter of time and effort – positive thinking, careful attention to diet, exercise and rest – before I entered a permanent and complete remission. Everyone around me was pleased to support this idea and even after I had been ill for years and the situation had deteriorated, my attempts to talk frankly of this met with pleas that I must not give up hope! Eventually, I noticed that my courageous outlook, my heroic refusal to admit defeat, was actually putting my life on hold. Meanwhile, I had to live with my spectacular failure to will myself back to good health. It took a different kind of courage to face facts and get on with life as it was. Recognising me as disabled was a big part of that. That is recognising the difference between my uncontrollable limitations and the limitations that I could actually do something about.

Levine *et al.* (1987) capture the therapeutic mixed blessing that can result from denial, which takes the form of disregard. Their study investigated the relationship between denial of illness and the course of recovery in coronary heart disease patients. Forty-five male patients, hospitalised for myocardial infarction or for coronary bypass surgery, were assessed for their level of denial. High deniers spent fewer days in intensive care and had fewer signs of cardiac dysfunction during hospitalisation, relative to low deniers. However, in the year following discharge, high deniers adapted more poorly than low deniers, by being more noncompliant with medical recommendations and requiring more days of hospitalisation. This suggests that denial of illness is adaptive during acute recovery, but may be maladaptive in the longer run.

Chattoo and Ahmed (2004, p. 24) tell of the enraged response of a young woman dying of cancer, to the involvement of a palliative care worker, as 'I am not having a Macmillan nurse. I don't need one. They are for the old and dying'. This act of denial, flying in the face of an awful reality, captures well what happens when we are so terrified with anxiety that a 'refusal to believe' defence is adopted.

From such illustrations, we can see that chronic insidious conditions such as heart disease or signs of cancer may not be seen as 'abnormal', provided one can carry on with daily life activities (Helman, 1986, p. 85). This suggests that illness is a disturbance of our social lives, with any perception that something is wrong, and guesses as to the cause experienced in a social context (Lorber and Moore, 2002). However, the argument put forward by psychodynamic thinking is that we must also consider the psychological dimension, with illness needing understanding as a psychosocial experience. The capacity to care for oneself, through self-monitoring and seeking appropriate help, lies in the ability to manage a self-care preoccupation about our distress. Such worry work and the ability to 'fuss about' (Winnicott, 1960) our health, originates in earlier parent–child experiences, where we have been the object of 'caring-as-worrying' (van Manen, 1998, p. 19–23). Prototypes about 'how to' and 'what to' fuss about when ill are thus internalised and then mirrored in our lives.

Any understanding of illness would be incomplete without considering the influence of racial and religious traditions. Whatever religious position one adopts, from sceptic to believer, all understanding begins with an appreciation of the meaning of timeless human predicaments. Race and religion have the potential to be a tremendous source of social and individual strength, be that in the belief of a good God, personified by concern, love and presence, or out of a racial identity, which invests the individual with a sense of uniqueness, community and heritage. Nurses need to consider how the patient's orientation to health/disease, is influenced by religious or racial traditions. As Chattoo and Ahmed (2004, p. 20) state: 'there is no way of living and dealing with illness outside the meaning ascribed to the illness within a particular culture'. This is a large topic in its own right and it is not possible to do more than introduce it here.

Regression is a defence against overwhelming anxiety, which leads to the adoption of assumptive world emotions, attitudes and reactions useful at an earlier point in development. The concept has associations, which are frankly judgemental. For instance, McGhie (1979, p. 151) describes regression as a 'less mature way of adjustment', with claims that as illness places individuals under stress, there is a 'tendency for patients to regress while in hospital... by becoming childish and over-dependent in their behaviour'. Indeed Guimon (2005) considers it normal for patients to exhibit a certain tendency to try to gain from their illness. Such secondary gain may be understandable and acceptable, when it is about seeking care and sympathy (for example, 'Man flu') and is in some ways an extension of Parsons' (1951) idea that illness is a socially sanctioned form of regression. Such critical perceptions possibly have their roots in the fact that regression is mostly observed in very young children confronted by anxiety provoking situations. For instance, the birth of another sibling may result in temper tantrums and behaviour such as enuresis, more usual in a younger child. Understanding regression as being drawn down towards a 'rock bottom attitude' as 'the only foundation for a renewed progression' (Erikson, 1974, p. 212) hopefully aids appreciation that both ill children and adults can be so beside themselves with worry, that they can get caught up in a rock bottom attitude, because they cannot articulate their distress.

Regression can become a malignant and self-harming form of relating to others, driven by needs for care and attention. An illustration is the repeated, anecdotal reports by community nurses of elderly patients whose leg ulcers fail to heal, resulting from non- compliance with treatment, accompanied at times with suspicions that healing is being impaired by deliberate self harm. This behaviour can be understood as a regressive act to maintain care and attention from the community nurses. In contrast, it is striking to note the finding of Benbow (2007) who reports a dramatic reduction in both non-compliance and post-healing recurrence of leg ulcers, with the inception of 'Leg Clubs'. Their philosophy promotes a social rather than medical environment, in which patients are empowered to participate, take ownership of their problem, and gain peer support from others in similar situations (Benbow, 2007). Such illustrations serve the idea that ordinary, ill people can engage in regressive self-destructive acts when they feel it is the only way to get attention. Therefore, part of the nursing task is to create conditions where patients gain concern and attention in a setting that promotes adaptive rather than the regressive actions.

It is perhaps best to think of regression as an inevitable feature of illness, which has the potential to be a destructive or adaptive, life-enhancing force. In their most benign form, such states of vulnerability and emotionality buy time to muster coping responses and find comfort within the misery of illness, by sharing feelings and fears within relationships of concern and conversation. Such enabling relationships, which allow the patient to engage in egocentric and self-pleasing activities, such as reading, sewing, listening to music, provide a platform of progression from the 'rock bottom' attitude. Such a positive defence mechanism can be explained as an extension of the notion of *transitional objects*, which have a root in parental encouragement for the child to develop its own soothers, in order to develop the capacity to be self-reliant, for example: 'Go and play...' (Winnicott,1958).

It is worth drawing attention again to the developmental fears prompted by illness, which have their roots in childhood (Strain, 1978). The earlier illustration from Sparkes (1998) about the athlete confronting the demise of the disciplined body-self provides a sad illustration of how serious illness can threaten basic integrity. Challenges to the illusions of self-sufficiency, indestructibility, and destiny-control, threw this athlete into psychic disarray. Illness threatens narcissistic integrity, the developmentally normal, sensual gratification gained from our body. It is always present and perhaps captured by the pains the majority of people go to, to look nice. It is not surprising that illness, which threatens the self-loving self, can lead to regression, a potential for interpersonal conflict, and inevitable distortions in relationships (Strain, 1978). Regression is also when distant memories and remnants of past relationships and experiences cause reflections in the present. For instance Muskin (1995) suggests illness can reactivate infantile wishes and fantasies for parental omnipotence (parents to be all-powerful and all protective), which are mirrored in distorted relationships with health professionals, with the patient wishing them to be therapeutically omnipotent, parental figures. Disillusionment can lead to rage, bitterness and disappointment. These are transference phenomena, described more fully in the next chapter.

A further developmental dread aroused in serious illness is a fear of loss of control of developmentally achieved functions, for instance, bladder control. Atwood and Weinstein (2002) suggest this is the reality for many elderly people, due to illness and ageing, leading to changes in family roles. For instance, the marital relationship may take on a parent–child dynamic when loss of control over elimination leads the care-giving partner to become responsible for changing and dressing, with the individual's dependency mirroring the experience of childhood (Schwartz, Bleiberg and Weissman, 1995). The ill person may be so ashamed of their lack of abilities that they withdraw, becoming despondent and angry (Atwood and Weinstein, 2002). Losing control over developmentally achieved functions can lead to decompensation in patients, whose esteem depends on a self-image unable to tolerate loss of control (Muskin, 1995). To decompensate means to more or less fall apart mentally and emotionally, when stressors are greater than coping abilities. Ageing and illness also negatively affect notions of the self as useful and attractive. Reactions to such changes centre upon key attachment relationships (for instance, partner or children) with the re-awakening of childlike worries about loss of approval, not being lovable or useful (Strain and Grossman, 1975). Forbes and Hoffart (1998) suggest that even when aged individuals have control over their care, the developmental dread of loss of control influences decision-making about when to use long-term care facilities to deal with increasing physical dependence. Their study determined that central to elderly people's thinking was a precarious balancing between their beliefs about why it was important to be independent and movement towards acceptance of physical care needs. Acceptance was 'making the best of it', in order to preserve some independence.

The experience of the aged who are ill, highly dependent and confused helps to illustrate how illness reawakens childhood anxieties and dreads. For instance, listening to the desperate, pensive cries of an elderly patient for their carer or long dead parent brings into emotional awareness the similarity of this response to that of a young ill child who is separated from a loved one. Such separation anxiety is a throwback to childhood when we knew we would die unless someone nurtured our needs. Triggers to such life-and-death-fears are abandonment, threats to adult relationships or loss of very important people and things, which define a world (Strain and Grossman, 1975). Chapters 5, 6 and 8 capture this beautifully.

Considerable research into a specific form of separation anxiety known as transfer anxiety has been undertaken (Robinson, 2002). This occurs when patients, particularly the elderly, are required to relocate from a known environment to an unfamiliar environment. Research studies of patient relocation over the last thirty years have consistently found that those transferred are 1.99 to 3.76 times more likely to die, when compared to those patients who are not transferred (Robinson, 2002). Robinson cites a critique of relocation studies by Horowitz and Schulz (1983), which importantly drew the conclusion that relocation mortality could be reduced by thoughtful preparation, which included preparing patients for transfer and maintaining the same staff before and after transfer.

As Strain and Grossman (1975) observe, health care systems make a remarkable expectation that patients will willingly place themselves and their trust into the hands of strangers. Health care settings are special environments, characterised by 'complexity, vibrancy and an ever-evolving organisation', which the ill person may find 'confusing, bewildering and frightening' (Muskin, 1995). Not available to patients is the years of socialisation and adaptation available to health workers, which enables them to inhabit and take for granted their environment (Muskin, 1995). Therefore, the patient has to cope with both illness and hospital adaptation while distressed. Admission involves removal from a safe and known environment to an alien, anxiety provoking and possibly painful context. Considerable adjustment and fortitude is required to cope with new regimes of ordering daily life, the strange faces of patients and staff, disconcerting noises, low levels of personal privacy and modesty, depersonalisation, and loss of body strength and competencies (Burns, 1991). Those socialised in health care culture can lose sight of the symbolic and historical associations of hospitals as fearful places, whose very odours convey messages of pain, suffering, death, as well as loss of control (Muskin, 1995). Such fears, and symbolic associations are continuously reinforced as shown by the current public preoccupations with hospital-acquired infection and cases of hospital-induced starvation. Therefore, it is understandable why the health care system can reawaken in patients childhood fears of strangers, with health staff viewed as having the potential to cause pain, neglect and disease.

Similarly, it is understandable why mutilation fears exist because of treatment for patients. Particularly when recognising the time span and 'heroic' nature of treatment regimes for diseases such as vascular insufficiency, leukaemia and breast cancer, with the frequent failure of repeated treatments. While it is important for health professionals to be able to envision as successful a treatment history that moves seamlessly over many years from cure to palliative regimes, it is understandable that the patient may view it as 'a rotten way to end up' (Murray Parkes

1975), given their journey of dread, pain, mutilation, remission, hope and relapse. This predicament was illustrated recently by the decision of 13-year-old Hannah Jones to turn down a heart transplant (*The Guardian*, 12 November 2008). Hannah felt she had 'too much trauma associated with hospital' resulting from developing leukaemia aged four, with successful treatment damaging her heart, leading to six cardiac operations, in attempts to improve its pumping capacity. Repeated hospitalisations inevitably result in patients developing a knowledgeable attitude both about their illness and towards healthcare staff, particularly, when the severity of illness causes dependence on others, leading to fears of vulnerability. Chronic illness casts a long shadow over all aspects of life as it initiates the requirement for a conscious regime of health maintenance and a self-consciousness emanating from a lack of spontaneity (Kelly and Millward 2004). It is hardly surprising therefore, that patients take a particularly critical interest in how others treat and care for them. Such patient predicaments about who controls what about their body can cause childhood dependency conflicts to re-emerge.

Conclusion

The intent of this chapter was to convey an explanation of responses to illness and loss, which recognises the importance of childhood experience in establishing worldviews of assumptions about our body, our health and what we do when we are ill. In an attempt to assist empathic understanding of patients, the mental defences against fears and anxieties roused by illness and loss are described and illustrated.

Telford, Kralik and Koch (2006, p. 457), following a literature review about illness acceptance or denial, offer a useful caution about an uncritical adoption of such ideas 'to categorize people's responses to living with chronic illness'. They identify the danger that health professionals may understand illness only within an acceptance-denial framework, not listening to the patient's unique story of illness. They argue for privileging the patient's experience, to develop a sensitive, focused response. It could be argued that the problem does not rest with the ideas, but with a narrow interpretation of another's experience by health professionals who only seek illness acceptance and compliance. Part of the problem lies in the narrative of health professionals who need quick and if possible, happy endings. Sparkes (1998) points out that little attention in the health-illness research literature is upon narratives about prolonged, fruitless struggles to reconstruct the self.

Nursing work is mainly about the 'brutal predicaments' of ill people (Koch, 1998). At its most bleak, though important, such work may be doing no more than to bear witness, so that the patient does not die alone. The sudden terror of anticipating death, certainly in war, includes reports of dying soldiers pleading for their mother (Hastings, 2007). Such primal screams speak to the importance and enduring nature of affectional and attachment bonds. Ways are needed to appreciate how early relationships influence responses when patients are scared and out of their depth. For instance, imagine the experience of total dependence on others when the only prototypes reside in the imprint of early handling. Knowing that childhood fears, for instance of separation and of strangers, can reawaken in illness, helps nurses to engage with patients in a developmentally appropriate way.

A theme of this chapter has been about how effective relating in health care has health consequences (for example, leg ulcer healing and relocation mortality). Wilson (personal communication, 1987), a psychoanalyst, was responsible for creating the first hospital setting within which it was possible to care and treat the family, including mothers, fathers and children, when there was a mental health disturbance in maternal and parental relationships. This innovation arose out of a realisation that health care systems should, where possible, support parent–child relationships, rather than treat disordered maternal care by separating the mother and the child. The aim was to reduce any distress and madness induced by the health system and its institutional ways of separating and relating to patients, thereby making it more possible to study and treat the maternal/parental–child dynamic, uncontaminated by iatrogenic problems. Extrapolation of this innovation to other health care systems would suggest that central to effective nursing is care, which privileges the relational and developmental point of patients, with regard to physical and psychological vulnerability and frailty, and ways of coping with illness.

The experience of illness and loss

Similarly to Telford *et al.* (2006), Abma (1998) suggests that people give meaning to chaotic experiences and persuade others of their perspectives by the use of stories, which with time get revised to contain new fears, hopes and insights. What concerns Abma (1998) is the impact of the initial story upon mental health professionals, who may use it to sustain professional practice, missing the new stories, so preventing successful rehabilitation. Therefore, it is the ability to 'hear the unheard stories', which can change professional practice. The Robertsons' (1971) research, managed to 'hear the unheard stories' of hospitalised children separated from their parents, by using developmental theory to describe and explain the emotional plight of the child, leading to profound changes in the care of hospitalised children.

In this chapter, serious illness has been identified as a major loss that can shatter life's meaning. This is not given up without fight or protest, leading eventually to a new life-meaning, tied in a helpful or unhelpful way to what was lost. Nurses, through their relationships with ill people, not only bear witness to this psychosocial transition, but must inevitably influence its course. The belief is that psychodynamic, developmental ideas about illness as loss can inform empathic understanding of patients and usefully inform nursing care.

References

Abma, T.A. (1998). 'Storytelling as inquiry in a mental hospital.' *Qualitative Health Research* **8** (6): 821–36.

Astrow, A.B., Mattson, I., Ponet, J. and White, M. (2005). 'Inter-religious perspectives on hope and limits in cancer treatment.' *Journal of Clinical Oncology* **23** (11): 2569–73.

Athens, L. (1995). 'Dramatic self change.' *Sociological Quarterly* **36** (3): 571–86.

Atwood, J.D. and Weinstein, E. (2002). 'Family practice, family therapy: a collaboration of dialogue.' *Family Practice and Family Therapy*. Available from: Priory.com http: //www.priory.com/psych/family.htm. (Accessed 1 August 2008)

Baker, L.M. (1998). 'Sense making in Multiple Sclerosis: The information needs of people during an acute exacerbation.' *Qualitative Health Research* **8** (1): 106–20.

Benbow, M. (2007). 'Diagnosing and assessing wounds.' *Journal of Clinical Nursing* [on line] 21(8): 28–34. Available from: www.jcn.co.uk/journal.asp?MonthNum = 08&YearNum = 2007&ArticleID = 1088 - 46k (Accessed 30 July 2008)

Black, H.K. (2001). 'Jake's story: a middle-aged, working class man's physical and spiritual journey toward death.' *Qualitative Health Research* 11 (3): 293–307.

Blumenfield, M. and Thompson, T.L. (1985). 'The psychological reactions to physical illness.' In *Understanding Human Behaviour in Health and Illness*, ed. R.C. Simons. London: Williams and Wilkins, pp. 48–59.

Bowlby, J. (1969). *Attachment and Loss. Vol 1: Attachment*. London: Hogarth.

Bowlby, J. and Murray Parkes, C. (1970). 'Separation and loss within the family.' In *The Child in his Family. Vol 1, International Yearbook of Child Psychiatry and Allied Professions*, eds. E.J. Anthony and C. Koupernik. New York: John Wiley, pp. 197–216.

Burns, R.B. (1991). *Essential Psychology*, 2nd edn. Oxford: Kluwer Academic Publishers.

Channel 4 (2008). *Coping with illness*. Available from: www.channel4.com/health/microsites/P/picking_up_the_pieces/illness.html. (Accessed 31 July 2008)

Chattoo, S. and Ahmed, W. (2004). 'The meaning of cancer: illness, biography and social identity.' In *Identity and Health*, eds. D. Kelleher, G. Leavey. Abingdon, Oxon: Routledge, pp.19–36.

Corbin, J. (2003). 'The body in health and illness.' *Qualitative Health Research* 13(2): 256–67.

Erikson, E.H. (1974). *Identity, Youth and Crisis*. London: Faber and Faber.

Forbes, S. and Hoffart, N. (1998). 'Elders' decision making regarding the use of long-term care services: a precarious balance.' *Qualitative Health Research* 8(6): 736–50.

Guimon, J. (2005). 'Neurotic disorders.' In *Relational Mental Health: Beyond Evidence-Based Interventions*. Boulder, Col.: Springer, pp.179–84.

Hastings, M. (2007). *Nemesis: The Battle for Japan, 1944–45*. London: Harper Press.

Helman, C. (1986). *Culture, Health and Illness*. Bristol: Wright.

Holroyd, E.E. (2003). 'Chinese cultural influences on parental caregiving obligations towards children with disabilities.' *Qualitative Health Research* 13(1): 4–19.

Horowitz, M. and Schulz, R. (1983). 'The relocation controversy: Criticism and commentary on five recent studies.' *The Gerontologist* 21: 229–34.

Howse, K., Ebrahim, S. and Gooberman-Hill, R. (2005). 'Help-avoidance: why older people do not always seek help?' *Reviews in Clinical Gerontology* 14: 63–70.

Kelly, M.P. and Millward, L.M. (2004). 'Identity and illness.' In *Identity and Health*, eds. D. Kelleher and G.I. Leavey. Abingdon, Oxon: Routledge, pp. 1–15.

Kivimäki, M., Head, J., Ferrie, J.E., Hemingway, H., Shipley, M.J., Vahtera, J. and Marmot, M.G. (2005). 'Working while ill as a risk factor for serious coronary events: the Whitehall II Study.' *American Journal of Public Health* 95 (1): 98–102.

Koch, T. (1998). 'Reconceptualising rigour: the case for reflexivity.' *Journal of Advanced Nursing* 28(4): 882–90.

Levine, J., Warrenburg, S., Kerns, R., Schwartz, G., Delaney, R., Fontana, A., Gradman, A., Smith, S., Allen, S. and Cascione, R. (1987). 'The role of denial in recovery from coronary heart disease.' *Psychosomatic Medicine* 49(2): 109–17.

Lorber, J. and Moore, L.J. (2002). *Gender and the Social Construction of Illness*, 2nd edn. Alta Mira: New York Press.

Lubkin, I.M. and. Larsen, P.D. (2002). 'Illness behaviour and roles.' In *Chronic Illness: Impact and Interventions*, eds I.M. Lubkin and P.D. Larsen. Sudbury, Massachusetts: Jones and Bartlett, pp.23–44.

Marris, P. (1986). 'The conservative impulse.' In *Loss and Change* (Rev. Edn). London: Routledge and Kegan Paul, pp. 5–23.

McGhie, A. (1979). 'Unconscious motivation.' In *Psychology as Applied to Nursing*. Edinburgh: Churchill Livingstone, pp.139–53.

Murray Parkes, C. (1971). 'Psycho-social transitions a field for study.' *Social Science and Medicine* 5:101–15.

Murray Parkes, C. (1975). 'Psycho-social transitions: comparisons between reactions to loss of limb and loss of spouse.' *British Journal of Psychiatry* 127: 204–10.

Murray Parkes, C. (1988). 'Bereavement as a psychological transition: processes of adaptation to change.' *Journal of Social Issues* 44(3): 53–65.

Muskin, P.R. (1995). 'The medical hospital.' In *Psychodynamic Concepts in General Psychiatry*, eds H.J. Schwartz, E. Bleiberg and S.H. Weissman. Arlington VA: American Psychiatric Publishing Inc., pp. 69–88.

Ouch's blog (2008), BBC – Ouch! Disability Magazine – Weblog Available from: www.bbc.co.uk/blogs/ouch/ (Accessed 22 March 2008)

Parsons, T.P. (1951). *The Social System*. New York: Free Press.

Robertson, J. (1971). 'Young children in brief separation — a fresh look.' *Psychoanalytic Study of the Child* 26: 264–315.

Robinson, V. (2002). 'A brief literature review of the effects of relocation on the elderly.' *The Hospital Employees' Union of British Columbia*. 23 September 2002, pp. 3–14.

Schwartz, H.J., Bleiberg, E. and Weissman, S.H. (1995). *Psychodynamic Concepts in General Psychiatry*. Arlington, VA: American Psychiatric Publishing.

Skew, P. (2005). Does having children make you old? – Telegraph.co.uk. Available from: www.telegraph.co.uk/health/main.jhtml?xml = /health/2005/08/15/hmum15.xml (Accessed 30 July 2008)

Sparkes, A.C. (1998). 'Athletic identity: an Achilles' heel to the survival of self.' *Qualitative Health Research* 8(5): 644–64.

Strain, J.J. (1978). 'Psychological reactions to chronic medical illness.' *Psychiatric Quarterly* 51(3):173–83.

Strain, J.J. and Grossman, S. (1975). *Psychological Care of the Medically Ill*. New York: Appleton-Century-Crofts.

Telford, K., Kralik, D. and Koch, T. (2006). 'Acceptance and denial: implications for people adapting to chronic illness: a literature review.' *Journal of Advanced Nursing* 55(4): 457–64.

The Cuardian. 12 November 2008. 'Hannah's Choice'.

Van Manen, M. (1998). 'Modalities of body experience in illness and health.' *Qualitative Health Research* **8** (1): 7–24.

Winnicott, D. (1958). 'Transitional objects and transitional phenomena [1951].' In *Collected Papers: Through Paediatrics to Psychoanalysis.* London: Tavistock Publications, pp. 229–42.

Winnicott, D.W. (1960). 'The theory of the parent-infant relationship.' *International Journal of Psychoanalysis* **41**: 585–95

Chapter 4
Passing on the blame
Louise de Raeve

Introduction

This chapter will focus on the ideas of *transference* and *counter-transference*. In this context, transference will be considered from the perspective of what the patient brings unconsciously into the nurse–patient relationship and counter-transference will be understood as the nurse's conscious and unconscious emotional response to the patient. It would not be nonsense to speak of the nurse's transference to his/her patients and the patient's counter-transference response but the examination of counter-transference is for therapeutic purposes and as such is located within the clinician. These are technical terms and their meaning will be explored as the chapter unfolds. Related to these concepts, is the defence mechanism of *projective identification* and this will also be explored. In addition to looking at the individual response of the nurse, consideration will be given to the ways in which organisations and groups of people working together can facilitate or deplete the therapeutic efficacy of those who make up that team or organisation. For these ideas to become accessible and interesting, the chapter will make extensive use of an illustration from practice, involving nurses and doctors working together. First, however, it is necessary to consider what *transference* is.

Transference

Transference

Hughes and Pengelly (1997) define this as:
> ... the range of feelings, conflicts, defences and expectations of relationships projected unconsciously into a current relationship (classically, with a professional helper)

but originating in other, mostly earlier, relationships.
(Hughes and Pengelly, 1997, p. 80)

In Chapter 1, there was discussion about projection, including the example of the young girl who claimed that all her teachers were useless. For the sake of illustration, it now needs to be presumed that she told them so. In so doing, it is possible to construe that for this young person, her teachers represented a maternal prototype; that they might have been expected to contain accusations of uselessness in a way which, whilst not agreeing with these accusations, would hold the feelings provoked in them (anger, hurt perhaps) with understanding, rather than retaliation. This construal would entitle one to say that the teachers have become recipients of a maternal transference from this student. This transference has several, complex aspects to it. It conveys a belief in the containing possibility of maternal-like individuals (in this case teachers) in this student's environment, meaning that the complaint is worth making in the first place and indicating some good mothering in the student's original background, as well as some respect for her actual teachers. From another angle, the communication includes an idea that maternal figures may let one down badly by being useless, even if on this particular occasion it would seem to be a gross distortion of reality. This, however, may reflect a truth for this student as an inner reality, namely some failure in the mother–child relationship in early childhood may have left this youngster with a mother-inside-her who feels useless. In turn, this may have resulted in a corresponding difficulty for the student to be able to cope with failure in an adult way.

Nurses, whether male or female, are commonly recipients of maternal transferences from patients. This is precipitated by the necessarily heightened dependence of patients and the 'looking-after' role of nurses in relation to this dependency. Doctors, on the other hand may receive more paternal transferences because of their more authoritative function in the team. For the most part, these transferences are unproblematic and simply serve the patient's recovery but difficulties may arise in health care where the current reality suddenly links to something that happened in a patient's (or relative's) early life, precipitating an extreme reaction. This can be bewildering for carers to encounter, as some of the case study chapters demonstrate, for example 'Joe's story'. Identifying transferences with accuracy requires repeated experiences to perceive a pattern and this is difficult in a health care context where the relationship between nurse and patient (unlike that of psychotherapist and patient) has not been established to facilitate this. Nevertheless, the idea can be useful to keep in mind when the responses of patients (or their relatives) to the nurses who care for them seem peculiarly intense, irrational or strange.

What follows in this chapter is an account of a way of working on a ward at the Beth Israel Hospital in Boston, Massachusetts. The subsequent analysis of this will introduce the ideas of *projective identification* and *counter-transference*, making it clear how these link with the concept of *transference* just described.

Working together: a scenario

Working together

In March 1989, the Beth Israel Hospital opened a fourteen-bed medical-surgical unit, called 7 Gryzmish. This unit was established to provide care for acutely ill patients with intensive nursing needs. From its inception, the unit also aimed to support the continuing evolution of a model of nurse–physician collaboration, in the belief that this would be beneficial to the well-being of both staff and patients (Pike, 1991).

> As the practice on 7 Gryzmish has grown, essential elements of effective nurse–physician collaboration have emerged. There is the open acknowledgement that nurses and physicians share a common goal: the health and comfort of patients in their care. Closely related is an understanding that providers are interdependent, not autonomous. Accordingly, collaboration requires that nurses and physicians share responsibility and accountability for patient care. (Pike, 1991, pp. 352–3)

The article makes it clear that people struggled to sustain this spirit of collaboration but what helped them to do so was the initial commitment they had made to it. Pike gives an illustration of a 72-year-old patient (Mr S) who was gravely ill, did not want 'heroic measures' and where a 'Do Not Resuscitate' policy was in place. His deterioration and the infiltration of an IV line, led to an attempt to establish a central IV line. This caused a pneumothorax, leading to the insertion of a chest tube, causing pain and discomfort. The distressed family asked for no further aggressive treatment, which was respected and the patient was given oxygen and morphine and died two days later. Pike states:

> The nursing staff agonised over the pain and suffering he [Mr S] experienced. We began to place blame, and among ourselves talked of the callousness, aggressiveness, and insensitivity of physicians...of their ability 'only to cure, not to care'. We felt anger, frustration, pain, remorse, and guilt. (Pike, 1991, p. 354)

What the nurses did next was interesting: 'They took their discussion out of the nurse's lounge and shared their reactions with their physician partners' (Pike, 1991, p. 354).

> Together they gained tremendous insight. They learned that communication is imperative. It had not broken down in this case; it simply had not existed. Clinicians were basing actions on assumptions and mind reading. There had been a failure to set goals for Mr S's care ... Importantly, the nurses in this situation discovered that they are not alone in caring. They learned that physicians also care deeply about patients, and also agonize over moral dilemmas. (Pike, 1991, p. 354)

Analysis

Analysis

A step by step analysis of the preceding scenario will now be undertaken, linking it to ideas of counter-transference, the use of social defence mechanisms and containment in institutional contexts. Three different meanings of counter-transference appear in literature on the subject and these will be identified as **(1)**, **(2)** and **(3)** respectively.

Passing on the blame

> The nursing staff agonised over the pain and suffering he [Mr S] experienced ... We felt anger, frustration, pain, remorse, and guilt. (Pike, 1991, p. 354)

These feelings, familiar to any nurse in any similar situation are reminiscent of the statement by Menzies Lyth (1988) quoted in Chapter 1, which acknowledges the complexity and depth of feelings that nurses have to bear in their everyday work. By some understandings of the term, this is the counter-transference **(1)**, simply what the nurse feels in consequence of doing the job (Heimann, 1950). However, this 'catch-all' concept glosses over some interesting and important distinctions, distinctions which have come to reformulate the contemporary understanding of what counter-transference means.

It is clear that the feelings of 'anger, frustration, pain, remorse and guilt' belong to the individual nurses in the story, but we could also surmise that different individuals would feel these in different degrees. The nurse whose father was of a similar age when he died two years ago, will be likely to feel differently from the young nurse whose father is alive and well. Our personal histories inevitably inform our reactions to the work, it is not in our gift to be otherwise and indeed this contributes to our capacity to empathise, but sometimes we over-identify with the situation and this can be a problem. Reality may be lost sight of by reacting emotionally to a different situation as if it was the same situation as the one we remember. This becomes a muddle and we lose objectivity, thus compromising our capacity to nurse. Writing about social workers, Salzberger-Wittenberg (1970) says:

> The case worker like the client brings to the situation expectations, fears and problems transferred from the past. For instance, she may see in the client before her some aspect of her mother and consequently feel herself still to be in the position of a little girl, unable to help this adult. (Salzberger-Wittenberg, 1970, p.17)

She goes on to say:

> The term 'counter-transference' was coined to denote feelings which the worker transfers from the past and

inappropriately applies to the client or his problem. (Salzberger-Wittenberg, 1970, p.18)

It is this sense of counter-transference **(2)** which includes the worker's transference to the patient/client that can '...impede patient care, particularly if the countertransference is intense, enduring and unrecognised by the nurse' (Miles and Morse, 1995, p. 45).

On 7 Gryzmish, the nurses felt 'anger', 'frustration' and 'pain'. Why? They felt that the patient had died in unnecessary pain and discomfort but dying, where there is any time at all to be conscious of the experience, is also reputedly a journey involving just such feelings and the pain can be both of a physical and emotional nature (Kübler Ross, 1970). It is likely that through caring intensively for this patient, the nurses became containers (see Chapter 1 for an explanation of 'containment') for some of the patient's feelings: that they were unconsciously projected into the nurses and unconsciously the nurses accepted these projections. This is the defence mechanism of projective identification. This phenomenon, however, leads to a different understanding of the term 'counter-transference' **(3)**:

> In recent years the term counter-transference has also been used in a different sense: namely, to describe the reactions set off in the worker as a result of being receptive to the client's transferred feelings. These emotions, in so far as they correctly mirror the client's, are a most helpful guide to understanding. Often, they give us a clue to the feeling which may have remained unexpressed. (Salzburg-Wittenberg, 1970, p.18)

Miles and Morse (1995) give an illustration of the usefulness of this view of counter-transference **(3)**:

> When a countertransference identification is understood, it can be used to facilitate positive patient care. For example, the nurse who feels depressed may recognize that he or she is identifying with a patient's sense of despair. Interventions can then be designed to address that patient's depression. (Miles and Morse, 1995, p. 45)

Morse and Miles see this as 'identification' but I believe it is more complicated, and is technically *projective identification*, unless the nurse was independently suffering from depression and even then projective identification might be still operating but it would be hard to disentangle and hard to decide who was projecting into whom.

Projective identification is the mechanism which creates powerful counter-transference experiences. It is not the only mechanism, as simpler projections (as described in Chapter 1) and identifications may play their part, but it is usually a powerful dynamic in the understanding of counter-transference **(3)**. It is not the same as the patient's transference but often serves to convey it. Julia Segal (2003) explains it very clearly, giving acknowledgement to the person who first identified this phenomenon, Melanie Klein (1946) (reprinted in Klein 1988a). In what follows, Segal refers to 'unconscious phantasy'; an illustration of what this means is to be found in Chapter 1.

> My own understanding can be formulated in two ways. For clients I describe it by saying that there are feelings people cannot bear to feel, which they may at times evoke in others. For those comfortable with the Kleinian concept of unconscious phantasy, I say that there is a phantasy that one can get rid of emotions or other parts of the self into other people. This phantasy can be played out in a very concrete way, so that the other person experiences a particular feeling ...
>
> The way the 'recipient' responds to the projected emotional state is very important, particularly as they are being scrutinized by the person 'projecting'. Unrecognized, it can be an unsettling experience and may lead to a counterattack. Recognized, consciously or unconsciously, and understood by the 'recipient' the phantasy becomes a communication; a possibility of recognizing that both can experience something of the same feeling. In this situation it can be 'handed back' in a modified form as a shared , contained, and therefore more bearable, feeling. The primary model is that of the mother recognizing and interpreting her baby's cry correctly and saying, for example, 'there, there, you are a hungry little one aren't you?' (Segal 2003, p. 154)

Nurses and their patients

As O'Kelly (1998) writes:

> Counter-transference should be assumed when the nurse has strong emotional reactions that differ from the usual; when she finds it necessary to talk to others about one particular patient; when she allows violations of usual boundaries; or does things that cannot be justified as therapeutic. (O'Kelly, 1998, p. 393, citing Schroder, 1985)

It can include somatic sensations such as headaches, weariness or nausea ending up in the practitioner (Hughes and Pengelly, 1997, p. 81). A related phenomenon is that the 'recipient' may feel quite convinced at first that the emotional state is entirely their own business and nothing to do with the client; 'mine' not 'theirs' (Segal, 2003, p.155). In current literature, there are some developments and different views about the precise meaning of projective identification and these are usefully summarised by Galatariotou (2005, pp. 29–30).

It can be seen, therefore that counter-transference **(3)**, is something of a double-edged sword when it is formed by the mechanism of projective identification. It can be a deep way of coming to understand another person's distress and it can lead to empathic emotional and physical care. When not identified, however, it can result in uncontained enactments by the recipient of the projections, which may be far from therapeutic. Many of the case-study chapters in this book describe the struggle that goes on to try to sort this out, both as reflection in action and reflection on action (Schön 1991). These chapter authors capture the painful honesty required to conduct this self-analysis.

Three understandings of counter-transference have been described above, namely:

(1) Everything individual nurses feel in consequence of their direct contact with patients.

(2) Only those feelings that nurses inappropriately transfer from their personal pasts to their patients.

(3) The 'reactions set off in the worker [nurse] as a result of being receptive to the *client's [patient's]* transferred feelings' (Salzberger-Wittenberg, 1970, p. 18).

Distinguishing between the last two ideas **(2)** and **(3)** is difficult but also necessary because otherwise the patient may be conveniently viewed as the cause of all the nurse's emotional problems. In clinical supervision, it tends to be easier to identify the possible projective element from the patient and harder to get to grips with the nurse's possible transference to the patient. This is because clinical supervision is limited by the necessity of respecting individual privacy and focusing on the work rather than the psyche of the individual nurse.

Counter-transference will be a theme, either explicitly or implicitly in all the case-study chapters in this book. It will be used primarily in the third and last sense described by Salzberger-Wittenberg 1970.

> In recent years the term counter-transference has also been used in a different sense: namely, to describe the reactions set off in the worker as a result of being receptive to the client's transferred feelings. (Salzberger-Wittenberg, 1970, p.18)

We began to place blame, and among ourselves talked of the callousness, aggressiveness, and insensitivity of physicians … of their ability 'only to cure, not to care'. (Pike 1991, p. 354)

Blaming others when we are in a tight spot is a very common phenomenon but there is much to understand here. First, the nurses were so distressed by what they felt that they could not contain it, something had to give and what one sees happening is an enactment – others are blamed. The nurses caught up in this would probably have felt justified and self-righteously indignant. They would have been unconscious of the dynamics at work. These however can be described as the defences of splitting and projection (to include projective identification). The feeling that the nurses seemed to find hardest to tolerate was the guilt, because it is this that is first separated from the self (split off) and then pushed away (projected) into the doctors who are then viewed as the guilty ones who can be legitimately blamed. That they would have been feeling guilty anyway, would make them a good target for these projections (see Chapter 1). Menzies Lyth (1988, pp. 64, 74) refers to splitting and projection as primitive defences. This is because whilst appearing in adult life, they originate from early infancy. Such defences, if used extensively in adulthood, interfere greatly with an individual's (or a group's) ability to face reality, and live creatively in relation to that reality.

Guilt in health care is very difficult to deal with. The motivation to be a 'carer' in the first place is usually based on a wish to do good, to help others. When we find we have failed in some way, we tend to give ourselves a hard time and what can compound this is the difficulty we may have in sorting out what we are realistically responsible for and what not. Death for the patient on 7 Gryzmish was after all inevitable, and whilst everyone might hope to assist a patient to have a peaceful and pain free death, this is not always in our gift, no matter how extensive our expertise. Unrealistic senses of guilt, which may link in all of us with infantile phantasies (see Chapter 1) and anxieties about our aggression, tend to be very persecutory because we may condemn ourselves mercilessly. This is evident in the language the nurses used to accuse the doctors: 'callous', 'aggressive', 'insensitive', but which would all have been silent self-accusations. Projecting these failings would serve to shore up a good sense of self and have the unwanted bad part put elsewhere. What can be seen on 7 Gryzmish is how these phenomena of splitting and projection operated at a group level and how groups will tend to use the nearest 'outsider' group (in this case 'the doctors') to project into. There are many illustrations of this kind of process (Menzies Lyth, 1988, Main, 1989, Zagier Roberts, 1994, Cohn, 1994). No institution or group would be without such an illustration. What was particularly interesting, however, was what happened next.

> Having made a commitment to collaboration, they were also uncomfortable with the outrage they felt toward Mr S's physicians. As colleagues they felt a corresponding obligation to address this conflict. They took their discussion out of the nurses' lounge and shared their reactions with their physician partners. (Pike, 1991, p. 354)

Pike (1991) describes how the nurses also wanted to learn from what had happened. One thing about the mechanisms of splitting and projection is that no-one can learn anything, since there is action rather than thought and one needs thought to be able to learn. Hughes and Pengelly (1997) comment that:

> At the heart of the difficulty of many disturbed service users (and others at points of crisis) is their inability to tolerate the experience of painful and intense feelings, which are expelled as soon as they threaten to surface by means of 'action' such as violence, delinquency, abuse or self-harm – or excessive helpfulness or intellectualising. (Hughes and Pengelly, 1997, p. 81)

They describe this as 'jumping over' the unwanted experience straight into action, which would include projection (Hughes and Pengelly, 1997, p. 81). Impulsive action is preferred to painful reflection, albeit an unconscious 'choice'.

The 7 Gryzmish nurses felt there was something 'uncomfortable' about their attitude to the physicians. This suggests some lingering sense that blaming them so completely was not quite 'real' after all. What the nurses were able to call upon to help them was the commitment to discussion that they and the physicians had made when the ward was first established. One can see here how large group agreements (which could be encouraged and facilitated by managers) can serve to contain inter-group conflict and permit resolution of the disagreement. In this particular scenario, this is what occurred:

> Together, they gained tremendous insight. They learned that communication is imperative ... Importantly the nurses in this situation discovered that they are not alone in caring. They learned that physicians also care deeply about patients, and also agonize over moral dilemmas ... (Pike, 1991, p. 354)

At an unconscious level what occurred was the re-owning of what had been projected. Once in dialogue with the physicians and seeing them as similarly human and struggling, it was no longer possible to maintain the rigid projection of blame. But the group discussion must have also helped individuals achieve a better sense of the reality of what they were and were not responsible for. This is because to re-own the projections, the persecutory feeling must also have lessened. Remorse is referred to and it seems it became possible for people to share their feelings of sadness about what had happened. They could think about their own and each other's contribution to this, without resort to blame. This sharing of sadness permitted further thinking. Efforts were made to understand why things had occurred as they did and what could be done to try and prevent the same thing happening again.

Not all groups are so successful in being able to resolve conflict satisfactorily, but one might say that what helped here would have been their shared history of trying to do so and their respect and affection for each other, plus perhaps the support and expectations of the wider institution surrounding them. In being able to find a resolution, they were (at a group and an individual level) able to replace the primitive defences of splitting and projection with more flexible and creative ones. Language is a form of symbolisation and in being able to put to each other what they felt, the enactment of the primitive defences simply became obsolete. Nobody would have decided not to do it anymore because it was not conscious anyway, but the necessity for splitting and projecting would just fall away in the new context, where discussion was offered instead. Achieving this, however, would have been painful. The language needed to convey such feelings is always struggled for and sincerity would have to be an essential aspect of the shared commitment. One way of describing what occurred would be to say that shared mourning happened and this led to an increase in symbolisation, thought and creativity.

Symbolisation is not itself viewed as a defence mechanism but it is intimately connected with sublimation, which: 'may be defined as a redirection of repressed impulses into socially acceptable channels' (McGhie, 1979, p.149). Menzies Lyth (1988) referring to the primitive defence system of the nursing service states:

> The social defences prevent the individual from realizing to the full her capacity for concern, compassion and sympathy, and for action based on these feelings which would strengthen her belief in the good aspects of herself and her capacity to use them. The defence system strikes directly, therefore, at the roots of sublimatory activities in which infantile anxieties are reworked in symbolic form and modified. (Menzies Lyth, 1988, p. 75)

In the illustration from 7 Gryzmish, the nurses had initially used primitive defences by trying to split off and project their feelings (push them out of their conscious awareness and project them elsewhere). In becoming able to fully own them consciously, through the processes of mourning and symbolisation, a more flexible and creative outlook emerged (the past was the past, what could they do now to change things?). This could be described as movement from a persecutory inward-looking position to an outward-looking, hopeful view of the world. This also illustrates movement from the paranoid-schizoid position into the depressive position, as first described by Melanie Klein (1988b) and briefly discussed in Chapter 2 of this book. Being able to symbolise is pre-supposed in this shift of position. The capacity to play in early childhood indicates the development of symbolic capacity. Certainly in adulthood, enjoyable engagement with theatre and cinema depend on the audience having a capacity to symbolise and to suspend disbelief. The freedom to play, if only with ideas, requires space free from persecutory pressure. Facilitating the capacity to mourn, to symbolise and to play creatively with ideas could be said to be a central task of supervision in any profession. Hopefully this then enhances sublimation and meaningful engagement with the world.

Other chapters in this book refer to some additional defence mechanisms. *Displacement* is mentioned in Chapters 6, 7 and 10 and *manic defences* are referred to in Chapter 13. At its simplest, displacement occurs when, for example, one is angry with x and takes it out on y, who is a safer target. An illustration would be kicking the dog, rather than one's partner. However, the mechanisms at work in displacement involve those already described: identification and projection; a situation is identified with, as being similar to the one that has engendered strong feelings, and then projected into, as if it was the same. As in the case of the dog, it can have regrettable and even highly pathological consequences.

Interestingly, however, in Chapters 6 and 7, the idea of *displacement* is used differently to explain empathy. Here it is not operating as a defence to be concerned about but rather as something to encourage. As Klein (1959) says: 'By attributing part of our feelings to the other person, we understand their feelings, needs and satisfactions; in other words, we are putting ourselves into the other person's shoes' (Klein, 1959, p. 295). This of course can go too far and nurses may then lose their professional boundaries, as Heather Davies observes in Chapter 12.

Manic defences are characterised by efforts to repair something but in such a way that the effort is omnipotent and quite out of touch with reality. As with the 'passing on the blame' scenario described previously, manic defences are another consequence of extreme anxiety and of being unable to mourn; they are also a defence against mourning. Such manic behaviour is exemplified in the 'fevered love' idea described by Alun Jones (Chapter 13) and in the ward observations described by Skogstad (2000). It is characterised by frantic or excited activity where the activity seems to have taken on a life of its own, as a magical reparative function which is quite illusory. Skogstad describes the way in which, after many deaths on the ward, the nurses became engaged in moving patients in the unit. He acknowledges that some of this might have been necessary but concludes that overall, it was excessive, sometimes counter-productive, and conducted as if, in the mere action of it, patients might be thought to be on the way to recovery (Skgostad, 2000, p.114). This would be 'magical' indeed.

Conclusion

This chapter has explored the concepts of transference, counter-transference and the role of projective identification in relation to these two ideas and in relation to group phenomena and social defences. Simultaneously, this served to illustrate moving from a paranoid-schizoid position to a depressive position, as described in Chapter 2. These, and other concepts identified in this theoretical section of the book are difficult to grasp. Hopefully, however, the next section of the book, the case studies, will serve to make them much clearer, by providing lots of illustrations. The seven chapters which follow are written by experienced nurses reflecting on their clinical work in the light of the theoretical ideas already raised. They make compelling reading, addressing sometimes mundane and sometimes very extreme and unusual experiences in practice.

References

Cohn, N. (1994). 'Attending to emotional issues on a special care baby unit.' In *The Unconscious at Work: Individual and Organizational Stress in the Human Services*, eds. A. Obholzer and V. Zagier Roberts. London: Routledge, pp. 60–6.

Galatariotou, C. (2005). 'The defences.' In I*ntroducing Psychoanalysis: Essential Themes and Topics*, S. Budd and R. Rusbridger, eds. London: Routledge, pp. 14–38.

Heimann, P. (1950). 'On counter-transference.' *International Journal of Psychoanalysis* 31: 81–4.

Hughes, L. and Pengelly, P. (1997). *Staff Supervision in a Turbulent Environment*. London: Jessica Kingsley.

Klein, M. (1959). 'Our adult world and its roots in infancy.' *Human Relations* 12: 291–303.

Klein, M. (1988a). 'Notes on some schizoid mechanisms' [1946]. In *Envy and Gratitude and Other Works 1946–1963*. London: Virago Press Ltd., pp. 1–24.

Klein, M. (1988b). 'Some theoretical conclusions regarding the emotional life of the infant' [1952]. In *Envy and Gratitude and Other Works 1946–1963*. London: Virago Press Ltd., pp. 61–93.

Kübler-Ross, E. (1970). *On Death and Dying*. London: Tavistock.

McGhie, A. (1979). *Psychology as Applied to Nursing,* 7th edition. Edinburgh: Churchill Livingstone.

Main, T. (1989). *The Ailment and Other Psychoanalytic Essays*. London: Free Association Books.

Menzies Lyth, I. (1988). *Containing Anxiety in Institutions: Selected Essays*, Vol. 1. London: Free Association Books.

Miles, M. and Morse, J. (1995). 'Using the concepts of transference and counter-transference in the consultation process.' *Journal of the American Psychiatric Nurses Association* 1(2): 42–7.

O'Kelly, G. (1998). 'Countertransference in the nurse-patient relationship: a review of the literature.' *Journal of Advanced Nursing* 28(2): 391–7.

Pike, A.W. (1991). 'Moral outrage and moral discourse in nurse-physician collaboration.' *Journal of Professional Nursing* 7(6): 351–63.

Salzberger-Wittenberg, I. (1970). *Psycho-Analytic Insight and Relationships: a Kleinian Approach*. London: Routledge.

Schön, D.A. (1991). *The Reflective Practitioner: How Professionals Think in Action*. Aldershot: Arena, Ashgate Publishing Ltd.

Schroder, P. J. (1985). 'Recognising transference and countertransference.' *Journal of Psychosocial Nursing* 23(2): 21--6.

Segal, J. (2003). 'Your feelings or mine? Projective identification in a context of counselling families living with multiple sclerosis.' *Psychodynmic Practice* 9(2): 153–70.

Skogstad, W. (2000). 'Working in a world of bodies: a medical ward.' In *Observing Organisations: Anxiety, Defence and Culture in Health Care*, eds. R.D. Hinshelwood and W. Skogstad. London: Routledge, pp.101–21.

Nurses and their patients

Zagier Roberts, V. (1994). 'Till death us do part.' In *The Unconscious at Work: Individual and Organizational Stress in the Human Services*, eds. A. Obholzer and V. Zagier Roberts. London: Routledge, pp. 75–83.

Part II

Case studies

Chapter 5
A personal experience

Lois Jones

Introduction

As an experienced Health Visitor, I analyse my own experience as a patient recovering from viral encephalitis, from the perspective of psychodynamic theory. The exploration focuses on attachment theory, grief and the meaning of illness. Some defence mechanisms are also considered.

My experience

My experience

I was admitted to hospital with encephalitis, receiving care in a neurosurgical ward before going to a rehabilitation ward. The illness struck suddenly and dramatically, with no prior warning. As a result, I found myself confined to bed, unable to move or speak. The following interaction happened while I was on the neurosurgical ward, receiving treatment to fight the infection. Though I cannot be certain of the day or time the incident happened, the memory of it is etched permanently and vividly in my mind. It has not faded.

A nurse came into my room for no particular reason and stated: 'When I next speak to you, try and answer me will you?' The words used were expressed as a question, but to me, there was no mistaking the real meaning. It was an order, a command, as though I was a naughty child, deliberately and consciously refusing to speak. With that, the nurse left the room leaving me with heightened, complex anxieties. She had fed my worst fear; that I would be unable to communicate verbally ever again. Asking me to 'try' made me realise how dependent on others I would always be, because all I could do, at that time, was nod. I believe she was unthinking, with no idea that she had made an assumption that I simply was not 'trying' and choosing not to speak at all.

Discussion

Discussion

During my long stay in hospital many incidents happened, causing various degrees of response in me. What is described above, however, is the single incident which has caused a long-term lasting effect. It stands out to me. At the time, the nurse's words were stark; they created a whole web of new feelings, centred on the fact that the nurse had an expectation that I could and should speak. To me, it was as ridiculous an expectation as it would be to tell a paraplegic to walk, or a blind person to see! These things were simply not achievable. Basically, my perception at the time found it to be a serious incident, because it pinpointed the huge gap between reality and expectation.

The feelings the incident provoked in me initially included uselessness and helplessness. I felt isolated, alone. I felt angry with the nurse, angry with God, the world, with myself. I was also conscious of wanting to be approved of as a good patient, and not a difficult patient. Later, I felt a sense of relief. At the time, my motivation was to seek clues as to my prognosis, though no one hinted at anything regarding the future prognosis or what expectations I should have. Therefore, what the nurse said was a relief. She must have been expecting me to be able to answer within days! This was a clue! I would speak! Later, much later, I discovered the nurse had no expectations for me or my prognosis, she simply said something inappropriate and insensitive.

Was she trying her best to coax me along by urging me to speak? Perhaps she thought she could. She was, however, entirely uninformed because I later discovered that the consultants did not think I would ever speak again. My biggest need at the time was to find other ways of communication, using a nod, pointing a finger, body language, but no one was able to provide this help. There is a possibility that this nurse was managing the situation by taking an aggressive stance, to trigger my fight for recovery. If this was the case, it was not made clear to me and I continue to believe that it was inappropriate. She could have read my notes and seen the facts and using her skill and experience of working with strokes and other serious illnesses, she should have managed the situation more appropriately. The nurse's comments at the time seemed brutal to me, but nothing would have been right, except my return to normality.

Along with my loss of speech, my mobility was seriously compromised; it was not known if I would walk. My right arm was paralysed, with no movement in any part. I could not move a finger or grip anything. However, these things did not seem so important; the speech was paramount. Prior to her words, I was in a state of despair; the process of loss and grief had begun. Lack of hope, lack of direction, lack of prognosis and lack of future prospects were all interacting, creating an enormous sense of loss.

This loss included the loss of what I was, the loss of my planned future, the loss of physical capabilities, loss of emotional well-being, loss of my intellectual potential, loss of my social skills, even the total loss of my established being and reversal of my status in all relationships. My status in the family, as mother of two young children, as earner, was all lost. I no longer saw myself as a working wife and mother, but as someone lying in bed unable to express myself, someone who was totally devastated, having lost myself and everything.

Murray Parkes (1975) notes that when a person is forced by illness to give up their view of the world, and their place in it, they work to replace this with another world view. Such a 'psychosocial transition', according to Parkes, follows a pattern of responses. This is the position I found myself in, recreating my own, new world view. It was frightening. My immediate response was to realise that my life had changed dramatically, a change for the worse. I now saw myself as a different person with a different perspective, one where I was in a wheelchair, unable to care for my children at all, and mute.

I was caught up in a 'process of realisation' (Bowlby and Parkes, 1970). I was faced with the unwanted prospect of rethinking my whole outlook on the world. This 'process of realisation', according to Bowlby and Parkes (1970), is one which develops through phases, which include a phase of 'numbness', 'pining', 'disorganisation' and finally a phase of 'reorganisation'. Bowlby and Parkes (1970) indicate that these phases are not clear cut and finite. Looking back, I now know that I experienced them all within a few hours of being struck ill. Reorganisation is still ongoing, and to a lesser extent, so are the other phases.

Amongst all this, I should emphasise that ignorance, through a lack of knowledge, lack of information, was central to my mental state. There had been a prognosis but it had not been shared with me, or any of my family. I worked it out for myself that no prognosis meant a very bad one, considered too bad to reveal to me and for me to accept. I was in mental torment as the lack of fact was, in itself, a 'worst case scenario'. My perception was focused on the gap between reality and fantasy: at that time, the 'fantasy' was the absolute worst-case, hence I was unable to move on and cling to any hope, since, for me, the reality was as hopeless as 'worst-case' implies.

At this time, my family surrounded me and comforted me, though I was aware that they were unaware of the prognosis. They believed I was suffering from some sort of strange dramatic flu-type virus, which, after it had been killed, would leave me weak: in six weeks or so I'd get up and walk and talk and return to my former self, and they behaved accordingly. In this information limbo, I had nothing to build on and I became frustrated, angry and grief stricken. There came a time when, on reflection, I badly needed to attach myself to someone or something, to give me some sort of security. I had a striking need to attach myself to something definite, concrete and established. I needed someone or something on which I could build a new me.

I was in need of a professional, independent, autonomous person outside the family, to form a relationship with. Such a professional person would help me accept and understand what was happening, and sensitively help me come to terms with my losses and future prospects. I needed to put my faith and confidence into a professionally inspired relationship and establish a professional communication.

In this nurse's defence, the situation was challenging for her. I was constantly surrounded by family and friends. From my own choice, I wanted familiar people around me and there was permanently someone at my side. Thus, I did not present myself in a way that encouraged new relationships to form. In my opinion though, this nurse had relationship choices; she could have chosen a social, informal relationship which did not become personal, leaving that to my family, whilst she tended to her practical tasks and ensured my basic care. Or she could have chosen to engage in a more intimate relationship with me, involving professional trust and confidence, a relationship where 'holding', 'handling' and 'object presenting' theories could come into play (Winnicott, 1988). Instead, she chose to offer some professional handling and holding by coercive messages to motivate me to talk. She did this without first building trust or confidence. It appeared that she assumed I had trust and confidence in her. In effect, the lack of these made it impossible for any 'holding' and 'handling' theories to come into play.

At that time, much like a baby, I had feelings of insecurity, fear and vulnerability. My basic emotional and personal needs were to form a new, strong attachment with a person of trust. I needed a person to hold me, handle me and help me to understand through object presenting, the new world and my place in it. I needed a nurse or professional to support me and help me accept the new me.

Bowlby (1969) states that in infancy and childhood, the mother's love is as important for developing mental health as are protein and vitamins for the development of physical health. The initial relationship developed with a primary carer (usually the mother) acts as a model for future relationships. This motherly love, or in my particular case, professional care, allows affectionate, or trusting bonds to develop. Bowlby (1969) suggests that psychiatric problems can result from an individual's inability to make and maintain affectionate or trusting bonds in childhood (or in my case, in the post-traumatic period). Hence I was in a situation where a particular kind of nurturing was needed. My trauma created such chaos within me, emotionally, physically, and socially, that I was at risk of developing mental health problems, which no one could have helped me with, as my thoughts and fears were locked up inside me. In an ideal world a health professional would have applied strategies to enable me to channel and express my thought and fears. It is easy to apply hindsight after the event, yet surely, I was not unique in my reactions and they are well researched and documented. Professionals caring for patients like myself are not in a new situation; they have the advantage of experience and are in a position to build bridges to help the patient begin the process of acceptance and rehabilitation.

Nurses and their patients

Miesen (1997) describes how a world that is frightening, strange and uncertain, with no structure to hold on to, as mine was, activates a similar behaviour pattern demonstrated by infants in a strange environment. Their behaviour can demonstrate feelings of uncertainty. For me, suddenly taken out of and losing my normal environment, I was plunged into a totally different, frightening new world. The feelings aroused had devastating consequences. To be ordered to 'talk next time I see you' left me frustrated, helpless and much more. My feelings of depression, despair, and hopelessness increased through the reinforcement of my fear and anxiety. Although Miesen (1997) was discussing the effects of developing dementia, there are some parallels with my case.

I felt that the initial bond had been made without a basic trust or understanding between us and as a result, there was nothing to build on. Without a 'good enough mother/nurse' to help me develop and lead me towards emotional health, my fears became overwhelming, and I was unable to rely on this particular nurse to be sensitive to my needs. I felt that she simply not did understand and was therefore ill-equipped to deal with me.

On reflection, it must be noted that there are challenges when patients are nurses. Crawley (1994) describes how nurses often have difficulty when communicating with colleagues who are themselves ill or disabled, giving conflicting messages as to their own role or the expectations of the other. Perhaps the nurse assumed, incorrectly, that because I was a nurse, there was already a professional relationship and understanding between us. In this setting, though, I was not employed as a nurse, I was very much a patient and the title 'nurse' was irrelevant. The assumption of a professional level of trust between us was incorrect.

At this time my feelings needed to be managed and contained through empathy and protection from a jarring experience; this could only have been achieved by understanding my needs and experiences and through professional holding (Rafferty 2000). This could have led to better fulfilment and emotional development, while at the same time, the nurse would have grown and developed to become a 'good enough' mother figure/carer for a needy patient such as myself.

In such a situation, the professional needs to support the patient in her immediate suffering by 'recognising and responding appropriately' to her unique needs (Rafferty 2000, p. 56). The understanding of this, often intuitive, response is generally considered to be an important tool in the practice of nursing (McCutcheon and Pincombe, 2001) but it is a very difficult concept to define. Usually, it is thought of as a skill, which has its basis in our feelings, knowledge and experience, which when applied to nursing relationships, can positively affect the quality of patient care and outcomes. It is considered to be similar to the personal knowing of patients that nurses have. Carper (1978) identifies intuitive nursing as one of the four ways of 'knowing' how to approach nursing care. Such intuitive caring has its roots in emotional intelligence and would depend on a carer's professional knowledge, skills, attitudes and experience, enabling them to develop a 'nose' for approaching a patient with complex and difficult needs.

As well as relating to family and friends, who seriously underestimated my condition and the difficulties of recovery, I needed the safety net of a 'practice' relationship with a professional and the space to learn to trust and to relate to that trusting figure. I could then use this as a basis for future relationships. Without this possibility, I was operating in a void. I, the patient, was in need of an attachment figure. This would have enabled me to express and explore my anger, fear and other feelings in a safe, non-threatening situation, providing me with a sense of security to help me to come to terms with what had happened. An ongoing relationship, with the certain knowledge that my 'good enough' mother/carer would be available consistently to support me in this traumatic time, would have facilitated my emotional recovery through sensitive 'handling'.

Rather than being seen as regressive (see Chapter 3), Bowlby (1969) considers that attachment behaviour is a normal and healthy part of human nature at all times of life (see Chapter 2). Bowlby (1969) states that an attachment figure helps to enable the transition through an illness and can help to overcome despair by making the world secure and less frightening. My inability to find an attachment figure during this early traumatic period led me to search for someone to fill the role. It was a speech therapist who helped me to fill the gap. She spoke to me as a whole person, not as a patient who had physical needs to be met. It is significant that the speech therapist's role was to enable my speech, help me to express myself, and help me to make sense of my world. In this way she became a maternal figure that I could emotionally attach myself to, just like a 'good enough' mother who helps her infant to master language. I did attach myself to her and her intuitive handling of me gave me the security I had been yearning for. I began to build on it. This therapist, employed to provide speech therapy, did not approach her work in that narrow way. She perceived me as a young woman with complex needs and used a more holistic approach, attempting to care for me, the whole of me, not a patient with speech difficulty.

According to de Raeve (1992, p. 99) 'the ability to give good emotional care … requires us to be able to acknowledge how human we are'. In my particular case, as a patient, I felt that I was able to relate to the speech therapist because she related to me as a person. She was not there to give me a narrow course of speech therapy, she related to me as a whole person, the therapy was secondary. Winnicott's (1988) idea of 'object presenting' was evident in my attachment to my speech therapist. She brought the outside world to me by regular speech therapy. The therapy was the technicality of speech therapy, but additionally she brought a more holistic therapy, by her intuitive caring and 'handling' of me. She was never deterred by my sadness. This illustrates that she could acknowledge those aspects of me without being overwhelmed. She demonstrated great skill by being able to allow me to express sadness, fear, etc. without taking them personally, as family members would have. She could believe in me as a person with empathy, without pity. She created an environment that I felt comfortable in. I accepted her as an attachment figure, enabling me to explore my feelings. At the time it was especially important because my family were very much in denial of my condition, holding on to the 'strange flu' theory and my subsequent one hundred percent recovery. They were unable to help me.

Even when not available for me, she anticipated my needs, providing me with equipment, space and a substitute to enable speech practice. My fear was my future speech. She understood this. It was implicit in her approach. This focus on speech therapy gave me so much more than the beginning of speech; it gave me a way to process my thoughts in a constructive way. She gave me access to props to aid basic communication. She encouraged my sister to adopt the role of 'acting speech therapist' during her absence, because practising speech patterns provided the focus and the safe environment I needed, to explore my feelings and my situation. It was only through this that I began to have the faith, confidence and trust that I could meet the challenge of disabilities, work to overcome the many problems and begin to make a constructive, happy, secure, lifestyle for the new me. She helped me feel sufficiently secure to start taking tiny steps forward.

Much of our behaviour is influenced by factors that we are unaware of (see Chapter 1). This behaviour can be explained as being unconsciously motivated (McGhie, 1979). The whole hospital was buzzing with the words 'there's a health visitor on the neuro ward'. The fact that I was 'one of them' made my situation newsworthy. Most of the staff knew I was there. Significantly, this could have motivated the nurse's words; all nurses are human and at times feel threatened. Perhaps this coloured her view of me as a patient, as professionals are often uncomfortable nursing another health professional (Crawley, 1984). This is, perhaps, motivated by feelings of insecurity, vulnerability, and even fear. Crawley (1984) comments that nurses will speak differently with colleagues and patients, indicating that different communication systems are being used. When the patient is also a professional, the result is that nurses are unsure which system to use. We could argue our boundaries are threatened when nursing another health professional and so it is challenging. It is difficult to allow other nurses/doctors to be patients, as such situations can make us realise our own fragility, even mortality, provoking feelings such as discomfort, uneasiness and insecurity. An important factor here is that the nurse/doctor will feel he/she is being examined for competency by the patient; we fear being judged or criticised regularly.

The nurse in question was the authoritative figure, yet I was a health visitor. This may have distorted the relationship because her authority could have been threatened because of my skills, knowledge and experience. A whole host of mixed resentments can arise that are hard to objectify. The nurse may feel judged by the patient because she is a health professional too. This can make the nurse defensive, and feel vulnerable and threatened. She might wonder is she 'good enough'? As the patient, I too, was hypersensitive and my sole motivation at the time was to look for clues about my prognosis.

I doubt the nurse was aware how hurtful I interpreted her words to be. My feelings were exacerbated because my own situation was so very new and strange for me. Perhaps her motivation in telling me to speak was an unstated understanding that my speech would return? Her way of telling me that I would talk? Unfortunately, however, she made a serious error because the prognosis, unknown to me, was that I would never talk again. But I can understand her need to protect me from the knowledge that I would never talk again. At that early stage, my language development was bleak. As it transpired, I did learn to speak again, but it is imperative to note here that I am indeed highly unusual. It was later identified that I had articulatory dyspraxia; something which is seldom seen in isolation. Usually, it comes with a range of other speech and language problems. The nurse could not have known this. At that time, the likelihood was that I would have a wide range of speech and language problems and, given that the 'assault' on my brain was described as 'massive', I maintain it was foolhardy to second guess the specialist and expect me to talk. I could not swallow!

Skogstad (1997) identified that nurses used defensive nursing techniques to deal with the anxieties produced by care work. The defensive ways identified could involve manic excitement, like an adrenaline rush, exemplified by constantly moving patients in a ward (without logical rationale or acknowledgement of the patients' feelings) or by referring to people as their affected body parts (for example, the 'appendix' patient or the 'mute' patient) and thus not appearing to see a patient as a whole. Such defensive techniques can become organisational defences or 'socially structured defence mechanisms, which appear as elements in the organisation's structure, culture and mode of functioning' (Menzies Lyth, 1988, p. 50) (see also Chapter 4). I was, I daresay, 'the patient who could/would not talk'. It is easier to deal with than truly empathising with the individual human being, which could be a painful process.

Menzies Lyth (1988) conducted a study on the nursing service in a large general hospital, specifically focusing on the social systems that nurses utilised as a defence against anxiety. The findings of the study showed that 'by the nature of her profession the nurse is at considerable risk of being flooded by intense and unmanageable anxiety' (1988, p. 50). The root of this anxiety tended to be the relationship between the nurse and the patient, as dealing with constantly ill patients can arouse a variety of strong emotions within the nurse, which is difficult to deal with. Menzies Lyth (1988) considers that the nurses' strong feelings have a resemblance to the fantasy situations that exist for all individuals, the elements of which can be traced back to earliest childhood (see Chapters 2 and 3). These are difficult and powerful emotions to deal with. Generally, nurses portray a certain level of professional detachment when dealing with their patients. This is necessary to a certain degree to aid focus of the work towards the patient. Unfortunately, nurses can overdo this level of detachment and distance themselves psychologically from the actual patients they are attempting to nurse.

In terms of my hospitalisation, I wonder how frustrating my needs were for that particular nurse. It must have been very difficult for her to nurse someone who could not speak. It must have tested her patience and some days she may have been close to losing her patience and 'snapping'. Handicapping conditions, like loss of speech, make others feel handicapped too. It alters relationships. This is hard for all to tolerate. I think, possibly, the nurse found the frustration too hard to bear and turned to blame the patient for it, as if the patient, I, had made a choice to refuse to speak. In other words, she could not, at that moment, bear the frustration and pain of the reality of her and my predicament. There was loss of speech but an inability, then, to use non-verbal means of communication too. I accept it was difficult for her, yet in relation to me, the patient, I found the situation wanting.

I can acknowledge the anxiety and stress felt by the nurse. This is an indication that there could be more guidance for nurses in supporting them dealing with challenging emotional situations. I suspect I made her uneasy and she was uncomfortable dealing with me. This is an important issue to bear in mind when dealing with patients. Many aspects of nursing may be found difficult for us as individuals, leaving us feeling vulnerable. Subliminal cues that we give, can affect the patient's reaction to us, which, in turn, affects the care given to the patient. It is important that we use reflection and clinical supervision to help us to deal with our feelings and so help improve the human reactions to care. In my case, the nurse's subliminal response was negative. Had she reflected on the situation, she may have responded to me differently, or provided me with a tool to communicate.

If we can attempt to understand the concept of transference in relation to nursing, it can enable us to make sense of our experiences and assist in our professional growth. According to O'Kelly (1998), transference 'is an unconscious process in which a person displaces feelings, thoughts and behaviour originally experienced in relation to significant figures in the past, to a current relationship' (O'Kelly, 1998, p. 392), whereas the unconscious response of the nurse to the patient is referred to as counter-transference (see also Chapter 4).

Transference is evident in almost all relationships but due to the nature of nursing and the positions that patients find themselves in, the transference that nurses tend to receive is maternal in nature (de Raeve, 1992). Evidence of transference includes patients projecting their feelings regarding a significant person on to the nurse, in such a way that it appears the nurse is the original person involved. Generally, transference comes to light when the current situation is stressful for the individual. This makes me feel like I was searching for a maternal figure, a 'good enough' mother who, as in the mind and eye of an infant, would solve all my problems, enabling me to feel secure and happy. Did I see this nurse as a person in her own right or someone with no real identity, a solution to a problem? My needs, in fact, were impossible to meet.

The nurse, too, failed, I believe, to see me as a person in my own right. She treated me not as a patient but as a 'nurse' with no really genuine patient needs. She responded to the 'nurse' and she was guarded and avoided the real issues, making a huge mistake in finally offering what I wanted to hear, that I would talk (according to the hidden agenda and contained in the 'Next time I see you, talk' sentence). Indeed, her unconscious thought was to urge me to do the impossible.

I felt the nurse was projecting her sense of hopeless frustration, which I can now understand on reflection. I feel she coped with her own feelings by projecting these feelings on to me. This made me a sort of culprit, a person who was consciously and deliberately withholding speech. I feel she was angry with me for my inability to communicate. In this situation, it would have been best if she had engaged in clinical supervision and talked to another nurse, doctor or my speech therapist. The only way forward for her, in that situation, was to find a way to help me communicate with her, which she did not do.

Crawley (1984) discusses the challenges for nurses, dealing with nurses who are chronically sick. The illness alters the dynamics of relationships. Crawley maintains that when nurses deal with chronically sick friends and colleagues, they cease to become friends or colleagues, taking on a more professional 'nurse' role. The nurse who has an illness or disablement is expecting a 'friend' to visit and may be looking forward to it, as a chance to share her anxieties about her condition with a 'friend who is a nurse'. The result is that both parties give conflicting messages as to their own role and the role they expect of the other, and the role-changes seldom synchronise, leaving both people feeling uncomfortable, confused and inadequate. I cannot, agree with this, according to my own experience. My social circle, made up largely of health professionals, continued to be loyal friends. Crawley does, however, acknowledge that discomfort, confusion and inadequacies can follow when relating to patients who are nurses.

Conclusion

Writing this chapter has been a very interesting journey for me personally, not only as a patient but also as a nurse. I have reflected on the scenario initially described and considered the behaviour and motivation of the nurse and reflected on my own behaviour, motivation and responses. By reading and learning and becoming aware of psychodynamic theories, I have been able to make sense and give meaning to an experience which disturbed me.

Seven years after the incident, I have recovered, living with some impaired mobility and articulatory dyspraxia. There is no movement in my right arm or hand; they are one hundred percent non-functional. Now when I look back at the incident which triggered this study, I have moved on. On a personal level, I have made meaningful a situation that I felt was senseless. I am able to view the incident with the nurse as an unfortunate slip of the tongue, yet it concerned me a great deal at the time and since. In the mental torment I was in then, that one phrase could have caused irretrievable damage and pushed me over the edge.

This chapter emphasises the importance of an awareness of the theories, and suggests that increased awareness will lead to more sensitive, more professional health care. I feel strongly that my initial training was lacking. Surely, all individuals contemplating a career in nursing care should begin by becoming aware that communication is a fundamental and a crucial aspect of care? Above all, it is clear to me that not all nurses can do all things, yet there should be available a specialist professional who is skilled in helping those who cannot speak. His or her role would be to develop ways of communication and to provide counselling, to enable the patient to express anger, frustration and learn to accept their predicament. In addition, providing some ground rules for associate staff might help them deal better with patients who cannot speak for themselves.

References

Bowlby, J. (1969). 'Affectional bonds: their nature and origin.' In *Progress in Mental Health: Proceedings of the Seventh National Congress on Mental Health*, ed. H. Freeman. London: J. and A. Churchill, pp. 319–27.

Bowlby, J. and Murray Parkes, C. (1970). 'Separation and loss within the family.' In *The Child in His Family, International Year Book of Child Psychiatry and Allied Professions*, Vol.1, eds. E.J. Anthony and C. Koupernik. New York: John Wiley, pp.197–216.

Carper, B.A (1978). 'Fundamental patterns of knowing.' *Advances in Nursing Science* 1(1): 70–5.

Crawley, P. (1984). 'Once a nurse always a nurse – unless you are a patient.' *International Journal for the Advancement of Counselling* 7: 261–5.

de Raeve, L. (1992). 'Nurse-patient relationships at night: a psychosocial perspective.' In *Nursing at Night: A Professional Approach*, ed. R. McMahon. London: Scutari Press, pp. 97–108.

McCutcheon, H.H.I. and Pincombe, J. (2001). 'Intuition: an important tool in the practice of nursing.' *Journal of Advanced Nursing* 35(5): 342–8.

McGhie, A. (1979). *Psychology as Applied to Nursing*, 7th edn. Edinburgh: Churchill Livingstone.

Menzies Lyth, I. (1988). 'The functioning of social systems as a defence against anxiety.' In *Containing Anxiety in Institutions: Selected Essays*, Vol. 1. London: Free Association Books, pp. 43–85.

Miesen, B.M.L. (1997). *Caregiving in Dementia. Research and Applications*. Vol 2. London: Routledge.

Commentary on 'A personal experience'

Murray Parkes, C. (1975). 'Psycho-social transitions: comparison between reactions to loss of a limb and loss of a spouse.' *British Journal of Psychiatry* 127: 204—10.

O'Kelly, G. (1998). 'Countertransference in the nurse-patient relationship: a review of the literature.' *Journal of Advanced Nursing* 28(2): 391–7.

Rafferty, M.A. (2000). 'A conceptual model for clinical supervision in nursing and health visiting based upon Winnicott's (1960) theory of the parent-infant relationship.' *Journal of Psychiatry and Mental Health Nursing* 7: 153–61.

Skogstad, W. (1997). 'Working in a world of bodies, defensive techniques on a medical ward – a psychoanalytical observation.' *Psychoanalytic Psychotherapy* 11(3): 221–41.

Winnicott, D.W. (1988). *Babies and Their Mothers*. London: Free Association Books.

Commentary on 'A personal experience'
Mary Paget

In her chapter, Lois conveys very eloquently the frustrations of not being able to speak, as well as describing an interaction with a nurse where she was apparently dealt with in a very clumsy fashion. As a result, this incident stands out in a very stark manner for Lois, as it provoked in her feelings of helplessness and isolation at a time when she needed support and understanding. Lois was just beginning to recover from the illness but was also just beginning to realise what she had lost as a result of this. Physical function was clearly an issue, but in addition, she was confronting the ways that her life had changed for the worse and was faced with the enormous task of building a new version of that life. All of Lois' hopes and aspirations had been affected, as well as her role as a mother and her career prospects as a health visitor. Added to this were concerns about not knowing what the outcome of her illness was likely to be. Any one change of this nature is considered to be stressful, so one can only imagine the stress and anxiety of the dawning realisation, that every aspect of life is about to change. It is reasonable to assume that Lois was in a state of profound grief for the loss of her previous life and also in a state of extreme anxiety at the prospect of rebuilding that life. Bretherton (2005, p. 21) cites a personal communication from Parkes in 1989, who considers that grief can be seen as a process which is aimed at establishing a new identity, rather than as a mere state of being. However, just as with physical pain, emotional pain can overwhelm the individual. When a person is in this position, it becomes difficult to focus on anything other than the pain, which clouds everything. Such unbearable feelings can last for some time. Most nurses are familiar with the stages considered to represent the experience of grief and loss. Kübler-Ross (1970) summarised these stages as consisting of denial, anger, bargaining, depression and acceptance. Lois herself identifies that she was suffering from a sense of despair, but what also becomes clear in this chapter is that Lois was also very angry about her circumstances.

This puts Lois in a very difficult position; after all how does one deal with anger as a hospital in-patient? Who does one become angry with and how does one express this anger? It would be difficult for Lois to become angry with her own family, after all they were not to blame for her illness and more pragmatically, perhaps, they were providing Lois with as much support as they could. As Lois describes it, they were surrounding her and comforting her. To become angry with the family might be to alienate them at a time when she needed them more than ever. A nurse herself, Lois would have understood the inappropriateness of expressing her anger at the nurses, who for the most part were also trying to help her. It is possible that this one nurse, rather unwittingly, provided Lois with a focus for her anger, acting as a lightening rod that allowed the anger to be grounded and expressed rather than held inside. Did Lois need someone to be angry with, in order to displace her feelings of anger, thus allowing her to deal with her own feelings and begin to recover?

On the face of it, the nurse's words do seem tactless and uninformed, but it is also possible to read a different motivation into her words. My initial reaction to Lois' chapter was that the nurse was trying to be encouraging, trying to adopt a rehabilitative stance, albeit in a clumsy way. At the time of this incident, no-one really knew what the outcome for Lois was likely to be. Although the medical staff were apparently concerned that Lois would never recover to any extent and would not speak again, this hadn't been conveyed to a number of people, Lois and her family included. It is possible that the nurse was equally unaware about Lois' prognosis and prospects and was trying to elicit some sort of reaction from Lois that would prompt her to speak.

Commentary on 'A personal experience'

As Lois herself identifies, her main motivation at that time was to seek clues with regard to her prognosis; she and her family were in an information vacuum. Not knowing her prognosis allowed Lois to imagine the worst possible scenario. In this case, Lois' fantasy was much worse than the reality, yet in health care many professionals excuse the lack of information-giving, on the grounds that the reality may be too difficult to bear. Lois' experiences would suggest that this is a misplaced concern.

Unfortunately, the nurse's words were interpreted by Lois as an order or a command. It is impossible to say whether Lois misunderstood the nurse's intentions when she asked her to try to speak, as the tone of voice cannot be represented on paper. However, Habermas (1984) in his theory of communicative activity suggests that in every communication there is an 'illocutionary content' or a subtext as well as the words that are themselves spoken. In other words, in addition to the spoken content, the speech itself expresses things about the internal world of the speaker. If this is so, then maybe Lois discerned that the nurse was conveying her own innermost frustrations; that she too was frustrated by Lois' inability to communicate. On the other hand, perhaps Lois interpreted the words in a way that largely reflected her own feelings. As Lois herself says 'nothing at that time would have been right except my return to normality' and there was a dawning recognition that this was not going to happen. This is all supposition, but what is certain is that at that time, Lois felt she needed someone to soothe and hold her, not a command to try to speak. She needed to develop a trusting relationship with someone who could help her manage her emotional turmoil. If one considers Lois' situation in conjunction with Melanie Klein's (1932, cited by Money Kyrle, 1984) discussion of the infant's developing states of mind, one can see that there are close analogies with the paranoid-schizoid position. In this position, the newborn infant is in a completely un-integrated mental and emotional state. The infant is unaware of time; similarly hospital patients lose track of time, or time seems to pass very slowly. The infant has no language with which to communicate. Lois too had lost her ability to communicate and had to rely on body language to convey her needs as a result of her articulatory dyspraxia. The infant's main sensations relate to being fed, bathed, or being talked to; in the same way, Lois' world had shrunk to a series of care-giving tasks undertaken for her. Finally, the infant has not yet developed any sense of the boundaries of its body, and similarly, Lois had lost sensations to parts of her own body.

Just as the infant is in an un-integrated state, so Lois too was falling apart and needed someone to trust, who could help her hold her emotions together in the same way as the mother holds together the fragile emotions of the infant. She needed the 'good breast', the term coined by Klein to refer to those elements that give succour and comfort. And she also needed to split off those emotions causing her anxiety and attribute them to the 'bad breast'. This is a way of disowning persecutory feelings and attributing them to someone else; in this case, the nurse who told her to 'try'!

In the same way, it is possible that the nurse too needed some help to deal with her own emotions. Menzies Lyth (1988) speaks of the stresses of day-to-day nursing and the need for nurses to receive some form of support in the role. Dealing with handicapping conditions, such as a patient with loss of speech, can make others feel handicapped too and test one's patience. This is hard to tolerate. The nurse may have been short of patience that day and found the frustration too difficult to bear, snapping at Lois and blaming her for her own upset feelings. In this position, the nurse would have been unable to contain Lois' feelings.

Luckily for Lois, the speech therapist took on this role and through developing a therapeutic relationship was able to assuage Lois' anxieties. This is comparable to Bion's (1959) cited by Isaacs Elmhirst,1981) thoughts that the good mother is able to receive the infant's emotions, absorb them into herself and transform them into some sort of meaning. In other words, the mother takes the infant's unmanageable emotions and makes them manageable. The speech therapist became an attachment figure and in a very literal sense, helped Lois to transform her thoughts into words as well as helping Lois to manage her emotional state. As Lois eloquently puts it, 'she was never deterred by my sadness, frustration, insecurity, believed in me as a person and empathised without pity'. This means that she was able to acknowledge those aspects of Lois' emotions without being overwhelmed. She could contain the feelings and help Lois to hold on to a realistic hope.

It is clear to see that Lois suffered a devastating blow to her

Commentary on 'A personal experience'

sense of self and who she was planning to be. Unlike most patients, Lois has been able to articulate many of her feelings about this with a great deal of clarity and insight. While many nurses are intuitively able to sensitively hold, handle and manage the anguish of their patients, there are many nurses who cannot achieve this and focus their attentions on providing physical care. This chapter provides insight into some of the interactions and tensions between nurses and their patients and some understanding of the importance of providing effective emotional care, alongside physical care.

References

Bion, W.R. (1959). 'Attacks on linking.' *International Journal of Psycho-Analysis* 40: 308–15.

Bretherton, I. (2005). 'The roots and growing points of attachment theory' [1991]. In *Attachment Across the Life Cycle*, eds. C. M. Parkes, J. Stevenson-Hinde and P. Marris. London: Tavistock/Routledge, pp. 9–32.

Habermas, J. (1984). *Theory of Communicative Action*. Translated by Thomas McCarthy. Cambridge: Polity.

Isaacs Elmhirst, S. (1981). 'Bion and babies' [1980]. In *Do I Dare Disturb the Universe? A Memorial to Wilfred R. Bion*, ed. J. Grotstein. Beverley Hills, California: Caesura Press, pp. 84–91.

Klein, M. (1932). *The Psycho-Analysis of Children*. London: Hogarth Press and the Institute of Psycho-Analysis.

Kübler-Ross, E. (1970). *On Death and Dying*. London: Tavistock.

Menzies Lyth, I. (1988). *Containing Anxiety in Institutions: Selected Essays*. Vol. London: Free Association Books.

Money-Kyrle, R. ed. (1984). The Writings of Melanie Klein. Vol. 2 (trans. A. Strachey). New York: Free Press.

Chapter 6
Visiting time
Mary Isaac

Introduction

A request that arises on many busy wards is when the nurse in charge is asked if visitors can come in 'out of hours'. Sometimes the relatives are advised to adhere to the prescribed daily visiting period, as was the case with Mrs Jones, an elderly patient admitted to a busy hospital ward. Both she and her daughter, Mrs Evans, wished to spend long periods of time together. In this chapter, I ask three questions related to the above scenario and try to answer them by taking a psychodynamic perspective. Namely:

- Why did Mrs Jones want her daughter to stay?
- Why did Mrs Evans want to spend long periods of time with her mother?
- Why was I feeling sympathetic toward Mrs Jones, her daughter and Emma, the nurse in charge?

The theory of attachment is discussed, to explain why Mrs Jones and her daughter may have sought comfort in the situation they found themselves in. Bowlby (1969) suggests that in illness each of us will search for the comforting presence of those we know and trust, and will feel troubled, unhappy and anxious, if for any reason they are not available. When considering why I felt sympathetic to all concerned, the unconscious mental activities of identification and displacement are discussed. Interdependence, the life space and assumptive world are also explored as a means of understanding the feelings that emerged and the actions taken.

Nurses and their patients

The scenario

The scenario

As the Senior Nurse, I had responsibility and accountability for the nursing care delivered to the patients. During my working day, I routinely visited the wards and the particular interaction occurred with the nurse in charge of the ward (Emma) when I was in her ward office. When the telephone rang, Emma answered it. I could only hear what Emma said, though it became obvious very quickly that the relative was asking what time she could come to the ward to visit her mother. Emma responded with: 'As your mother has improved it would be better if you come at visiting time, as there is no need to stay for long periods now during the day.' There was more dialogue by the relative that I could not hear and Emma finished by saying: 'There is no need to come up early, your mother is settled and will be fine until this evening.' The conversation ended and the telephone was replaced.

I was rather surprised by the approach taken by Emma. I did not feel very comfortable with her response, as it brought back memories of asking to visit my grandmother outside of visiting times, and of the disappointment when the ward staff sometimes refused. As a result, I thought it was rather sad the daughter was put off visiting her mother, although I knew nothing at this stage about mother or daughter.

When the call was over, I asked: 'Who was on the phone?' Emma said that it was Mrs Jones' daughter and proceeded to give me some history. Mrs Jones had been admitted two days earlier for investigations. On admission she was very distressed and wanted her daughter to stay with her. Her daughter, Mrs Evans, stayed until 8pm that evening and then returned the next day about 10am, again staying until the evening. On the first night in hospital, Mrs. Jones had called for her daughter a number of times and told the nurses to leave her alone, but the second night she had called for her less often.

Today, Emma thought that Mrs Jones was better and therefore her daughter did not have to stay. I learned that Mrs Jones was eighty-four years old, living with her daughter who was her main carer. I said, 'It would be nice if Mrs Evans could come in today now her mother is feeling better,' but Emma thought it better if she now kept to the visiting hours because of the ward activity, for example, doctors rounds etc. I asked her to think about her decision, recounting an example of how, when my grandmother was in hospital, we wanted a member of the family to keep her company in the day, as we knew this would make her happier and she was likely to also eat and drink more for us, than for the nurses. Emma agreed to give this some thought.

Why did Mrs Jones want her daughter to stay?

Mrs Jones' wishes

Blumenfield and Thompson (1985) suggest that when a person has a physiological illness, there is also a psychological response. The first response to the illness experience is often apprehension or anxiety. Many factors determine the psychological response and one of these is the special meaning of this illness, which in this case is hospitalisation.

When patients are admitted to hospital they frequently feel anxious (Blumenfield and Thompson, 1985) as being admitted with an illness is usually seen as a significant event; the illness is perceived as potentially more serious than one that permits the patient to remain at home. To the patient, illness which results in admission to hospital can also mean the loss of function and strength (both physical and mental) by having to stay in bed or by not doing the usual daily things, such as working, cooking or shopping. This indicates a fear-provoking situation, fraught with danger, as we all like to believe we are self-sufficient and in control of what is happening to us. The hospital environment removes both. Illness can provoke a fear of strangers, as it can be frightening to put one's life into the hands of total strangers in a hospital setting. Illness can also mean fear of separation from the loving family, as a result of admission to hospital. It is important that we try and understand the anxiety and fears provoked in patients as a result of hospitalisation and assist them to reduce such fears.

It is suggested by de Raeve (1992) that time must be given to patients to provide psychological and emotional care. Therefore, it is just as important to be with patients as to be doing for patients. It is probably not reasonable for Mrs Jones' daughter to be at her mother's bedside day and night, while she is in hospital (after all they both need to rest sometimes) but, by being present, Mrs Evans is providing her mother with psychological care. In the reality of a busy surgical ward, there is little time for nurses to sit with patients for more than a few minutes during a span of duty, due to the overall level of necessary physical care. At night though, when most patients are settled and sleeping, it may be beneficial to sit at the bedside of a patient like Mrs Jones, who is calling out for her daughter. Doing this may help to prevent emotional distress and aid recovery and also be an economical use of the nurse's time, if it saves disruption later. I can remember the occasional patient who, shortly after the lights went down would start calling out and try to get out of bed. Sometimes, as a result of sitting with them, perhaps holding their hand or just being there at their bedside, they would settle and eventually sleep. There was nothing to actually do physically at this time, it was purely about being with them. Importantly, it was about looking after their psychological needs rather than their physical needs.

Mrs Jones had lived with her daughter for the past five years. Her health was deteriorating and she was gradually becoming more dependent. It is reasonable to presume a relationship of attachment was present between mother and daughter. Hazen and Shaver (1987) suggest attachment theory is a means to describe and explain people's enduring patterns of relationship from birth to death. Attachment was first studied in non-human animals, then in human infants and later in adults. When a human infant is separated from its parent, the infant goes through a series of three emotional reactions: the first is protest, in which the infant cries and refuses to be consoled by others, the second is despair, in which the infant is sad and passive and the third reaction is one of detachment, in which the infant actively disregards and avoids the parent on return. Farley and Shaver (2000) suggest that an attachment bond is marked by the tendency for a person to remain in close contact with the attachment figure and, when separation occurs, for there to be a degree of distress or protest. In times of illness, attachment figures are used as protection and support and to promote feelings of security and confidence. Bowlby (1969, p. 323) suggests that attachment is not only confined to the young. He suggests that in illness, each of us will search for the comforting presence of those we know and trust and will feel troubled, unhappy and anxious, if for any reason they are not available.

Visiting time

When Mrs Jones was admitted to hospital she was described as distressed and asking for her daughter. Her daughter stayed throughout the day and into the evening and Mrs Jones was calm. But in the night, particularly the first night, she was heard to be calling frequently for her daughter and telling the nurses to leave her alone. This behaviour could be seen as a protest at being separated from her daughter. It is possible that Mrs Jones was displaying similar responses to those Hazen and Shaver (1987) describe, as emotional reactions human infants go through when separated from a parent. It is important to emphasise the phase of protest indicates the belief that something might change. The more Mrs Jones protests, the more she may believe that her daughter will stay.

Mrs Jones' distress could also be attributed to being left alone in a strange environment. Bowlby (1969) identified the need for infants and small children to remain in proximity to the mother figure as a source of security and this need is enhanced when confronted with a strange situation or environment. The absence of the mother figure can trigger feelings of insecurity and distress. It is possible to draw an analogy with Mrs Jones' behaviour. Hospital is both a strange and unfamiliar environment; indeed Mrs Jones' surrounding world had completely changed. When her daughter left, Mrs Jones may have experienced strong feelings of insecurity, leading her to call out in her distress. When someone is ill, as in the case of Mrs Jones, it is reasonable to presume that she would seek comfort and security from her daughter and therefore become more settled when she was present.

Mrs Jones and her daughter appear to have had a good relationship, with a special bond between them. Therefore, in hospital, Mrs Jones may have been experiencing a depressive anxiety which Terry (1997) suggests can be especially provoked by experiences of loss and separation. This is also why she may have been protesting when her daughter was not present initially and became comforted when her daughter returned. Bowlby (1969) also points out that at each phase of our lives, we develop strong bonds to a few special individuals. When these bonds are intact, we feel secure and when the bonds are broken through separation or death, we become anxious or distressed. Mrs Jones and her daughter, in all probability, had this affectionate bond and this may be why Mrs Jones asked for her daughter to stay. For Mrs

Jones, her daughter's presence ensured the bond was maintained and as a result, she felt more secure and happier. Patients who are ill can feel vulnerable and powerless. Caring nurses need to recognise their vulnerability and aim to meet the patient's needs, a view supported by Nichols (1993).

The other consideration that needs to be taken into account is the psychological effect the hospital admission and the illness had on Mrs Jones. She had been admitted for investigations. Often when patients are admitted for investigations, they think all sorts of things, often fearing the worst possible outcome, such as fear of undergoing surgery, inoperable cancer or even death (see Chapter 3 for an elaboration of this). Nichols (1993) suggests that often, when patients are admitted for investigations, there is psychological distress and there is an important relationship between psychological state and recovery from illness. An example of this can be when a patient fails to comply with necessary treatment for their best chance of recovery, such as not taking their medication or not eating. Nichols (1993) suggests that when patients are low in morale or emotionally disturbed, they can jeopardise their recovery by abandoning the behaviours that give them the best chance. There is, however, no indication that Mrs Jones failed to comply with her treatment.

Mrs Jones was, in all probability, feeling frightened and as a result behaved at least initially, in such a way as to protect herself, for example, by calling out for her daughter. This action may be because the patient's 'safety system', that is to take flight or to fight, was activated, as a result of not knowing where her daughter was or in response to being in an unfamiliar environment, or because she was afraid she may need surgery (Cheston and Bender, 1999, p.133).

Why did the daughter want to spend time with her mother?

Mrs Evans' wishes

As I never actually asked Mrs Jones' daughter why she wanted to spend time on the ward with her mother, I can only make some assumptions. Namely, they were close, had a good relationship, with the daughter now caring for her mother as her mother's health gradually deteriorated. Chambers *et al.* (2001) suggest that often the carer's commitment to their relative is more than a duty. The carer has a strong emotional bond with their relative; this, combined with their in-depth knowledge of the person over many years, enables them to provide a high standard of personal care, which an institution could not match.

The attachment Mrs Jones felt toward her daughter was presumably reciprocated. Bowlby and Murray Parkes (1970) remind us that anxiety and distress can be caused by separations from loved ones. It is reasonable to presume her daughter was experiencing similar anxiety and distress. The illness of an elderly parent often brings about fear that one may be losing them. We understand that they are getting older and often frail in their advancing years, facing increasing difficulty in fighting off illness, but the realisation that death may be nearing brings increased anxiety. To most people, death means the loss of those whom we love (Blumenfield and Thompson, 1985). This may have been why Mrs Evans wanted to come and visit her mother for as long as possible each day. She may have been fearful her mother would not recover sufficiently to return home or may even have thought her mother might die. Bowlby (1969) suggests it is common knowledge that affectionate bonds and subjective states of strong emotion go together.

Mrs Evans was the main carer for her mother. Often when the carer is separated from the dependent person, they find the change difficult, both physically and emotionally (Cheston and Bender, 1999, p. 223). Mrs Evans could desire to be with her mother as a result of guilty feelings. She may feel that she failed her mother in some way, resulting in illness and hospital admission. It could simply be because she was trying to fill in the time until her mother was well enough to return home. In a study undertaken by Chambers et al. (2001) there was unanimous agreement amongst carers that caring was a twenty-four hour activity which was exhausting, but carers had learned to accept the disabilities and illnesses of their relatives and the resultant changes to their lives, and get on with it. Admission of the loved one to hospital often leaves the carer with unaccustomed time on their hands, during which anxieties can multiply.

Mrs Evans may also have wanted to be involved with planning and helping the professionals with her mother's care, to reduce the loss she felt from the separation, a view supported by Nichols

(1993). Carers remarked in the study undertaken by Chambers *et al.* (2001) that their relatives often had requirements which fell under the domain of nursing, covering the 'activities of daily living', for example, washing and dressing, giving medication and keeping them company. If this was something Mrs Evans was used to doing for her mother every day, it is understandable that she might wish to continue to provide some of this care and not have her role undervalued by professional carers. The shared perspective of professional and family carers is vital for the provision of quality care (Chambers *et al.* 2001). This requires good communication and mutual understanding.

Emma's perspective

Emma's perspective

Emma may have thought it was not convenient to have relatives on the ward constantly, due to the ongoing activity, like doctors' rounds and theatre sessions and the confidentiality requirements surrounding these activities. However, as someone whose own mother and grandmother had a very close relationship, I can perhaps appreciate how important it might be to Mrs Evans to maintain contact with her mother throughout the day and the need, therefore, to find a compromise. Emma may also think Mrs Evans needed a rest and should take this opportunity to have a break, but it is possible the daughter would not share this view. As many of us can acknowledge, it is difficult to rest when one is worried about someone who is close to one. Cheston and Bender (1999) express the view that if the ward staff undertake all the care and leave family carers without a role, this could damage a relationship just when both need it the most. Therefore, it is important the ward staff remember Mrs Jones will not be hospitalised indefinitely and that the daughter will resume the care of her mother. It is crucial the ward staff do not inadvertently damage the bond the mother and daughter have. We know carers have requested that nurses and other health care professionals be more aware of their needs and experiences and that they view hospital nurses as being in an ideal position to meet carers, provide support, offer advice and encourage involvement in the decision-making process (Chambers *et al.* 2001).

Why was I feeling sympathetic towards Mrs Jones, her daughter and Emma?

I am not certain why I felt sympathetic towards Mrs Jones and her daughter when I happened to hear the phone call. I remember feeling puzzled that Emma had taken this stance, thinking it was a pity she was taking this approach. I remember feeling sad that Mrs Evans had been told not to come in, thinking that if I had taken this call, I would have let her come. It stirred memories within me of when my own family members were in hospital and how as a family we liked to visit them frequently.

When I worked as a Sister, I often used to be flexible with visiting times and was never comfortable insisting that visitors should be confined to official times. When my own relatives were in hospital, I would often ask if I could call in for half an hour, outside of visiting time, and I know it meant a great deal to them as well as to me. This was due to the family relationship we had. Consequently, if relatives asked to visit, I tried to accommodate them. Over the last few years, I had not really heard any of the nurses I worked with be so rigid with relatives over visiting. I had only worked with Emma for a few weeks and I was not sure why she had this approach. Because I did not feel comfortable with her decision, I attempted to get her to change her mind, using my personal experience as an example.

McGhie (1979) suggests the mind can be divided into the conscious and the unconscious, with a barrier in between (see Chapter 1). There are many unconscious mental activities that can determine the way we behave. In my case it may be that I enacted a displacement response. Displacement, McGhie (1979) suggests, is the redirection of feelings from their source on to a substitute object. Displacement can allow the individual to release repressed feelings by displacing them on to another. It could be that my attitude to Mrs Jones and her daughter contained some elements transferred from my relationship with my family, in particular, a response to the hospitalisation of close relatives. My experience of being a relative and the way I was treated influenced how I wanted Mrs Jones and her daughter to be treated. I prefer to treat people in the way I wish to be treated myself, while acknowledging there is often a need to be sensitive to the subtle differences of the situations people find themselves in.

Beauchamp and Childress (2001) suggest that kindness; warmth and compassion are human qualities that are valued. I believed Emma would demonstrate these if she allowed Mrs Evans in to visit her mother during the day. Demonstrating such individualised sensitivity often generates an internal conflict for nurses, between getting the job done and meeting patients' emotional needs. When talking to ward nurses, they will tell you how busy the ward is and they are. They will give numerous examples of the direct practical care they are providing and the time it takes to undertake certain tasks. As Nichols (1993) identified, rarely do they go into detail about the level of emotional care a patient requires.

My role is essentially one of leadership, which includes using a range of leadership styles to get the best out of the staff I work with, a view supported by Pencheon and Koh (2000). I try to treat people with respect and give them responsibility, which according to Bryman (1996) are both qualities that a leader requires. In this situation, I believed it to be inappropriate to interrupt the telephone conversation, to assert my authority. I decided to use an empathic approach, following completion of the phone call, to invite Emma to reflect on the decision she had made. Therefore, drawing on my personal experience as a relative, I explained to Emma how it may feel to be told one is not able to come and visit one's mother all day, especially when the relationship is a close one. It may be that Emma had not had similar experiences. Perhaps if she had, she may not have been so quick to turn down Mrs Evans' request.

It is clear I was attempting to get Emma to change her mind because I did not agree with her. Why then did I not just use my position of authority and tell her to let Mrs Jones' daughter come and visit in the day? There are a number of reasons for this, the main one being I wanted to deal with this sensitively, not wanting to undermine the decision she had made. I had recently taken over responsibility for this clinical area and Emma had commenced taking charge of the ward after a period of absence. It was important to build a team that could work together and take things forward. If I were to insist upon having my own way every time I did not agree with a decision she made, then I would be very shortsighted and achieve nothing in the long term. To take this ward and the staff forward, it was important to maintain good relationships and make well-balanced judgements. Covey (1999) points out the importance of recognising the need for interdependence. Interdependence he suggests is:

> … far more mature than dependence or independence. If I am interdependent I am self reliant and capable, but I also realise that you and I working together can accomplish far more than even at my best I could accomplish alone. (Covey 1999, p. 51)

Bearing interdependence in mind, I was hoping to get Emma to change her mind through discussion rather than by insistence. In fact I had decided very early on in this encounter not to insist, as I thought it might damage our early relationship.

Conclusion

The situation of a relative phoning up to visit outside of visiting hours is a fairly common occurrence. However, it is more unusual not to come to some sort of compromise when a relative asks to visit outside of the designated times. It would have been easy for me to just say: 'Let Mrs Evans in to visit her mother,' when I was in the office with Emma but I believed it would be more appropriate for her to reflect on the decision she had made. Therefore, the approach to encourage Emma to change her mind, through the use of a personal example, was justified in this case. It is worth noting that later in the day, when I returned to the ward, Mrs Evans was there visiting her mother and helping her eat a snack she had brought in for her. Although I am not sure if she was there as a direct result of my request to Emma to reconsider, the main thing as far as I was concerned was that Mrs Evans was there with her mother.

References

Beauchamp, T.L. and Childress, J.F. (2001). *Principles of Biomedical Ethics*, 5th edn. New York: Oxford University Press Inc.

Blumenfield, M. and Thompson, T.L. (1985). 'The psychological reactions to physical illness.' In *Understanding Human Behaviour in Health and Illness*, ed. R.C. Simons, 3rd edn. London: Williams and Wilkins, pp. 48–59.

Bowlby, J. (1969). 'Affectional bonds: their nature and origin.' In *Progress in Mental Health: Proceedings of the Seventh International Congress on Mental Health*, ed. H. Freeman. London: J. and A. Churchill, pp. 319–27.

Bowlby, J. and Murray Parkes, C. (1970). 'Separation and loss within the family.' In *The Child in his Family: International Yearbook of Child Psychiatry and Allied Professions*, Vol. 1, eds. E.J. Anthony and C. Koupernik. New York: John Wiley, pp. 197–216.

Bryman, A. (1996). 'Leadership in organisations.' In *Handbook of Organisation Studies*, eds. S.R. Clegg, C. Hardy and W.R. Nord. London: Sage, pp. 276–92.

Chambers, M., Ryan, A.A. and Connor, L. (2001). 'Exploring the emotional support needs and coping strategies of family carers.' *Psychiatric and Mental Health Nursing* **8** (2): 99–106.

Cheston, R. and Bender, M. (1999). *Understanding Dementia*. London: Jessica Kingsley.

Covey, S. R. (1999). The 7 Habits of Highly Effective People. London: Simon and Schuster UK Limited.

de Raeve, L. (1992). 'Nurse-patient relationships at night: a psychosocial perspective.' In *Nursing at Night: A Professional Approach*, ed. R. McMahon. London: Scutari Press, pp. 97–108.

Farley, R.C. and Shaver, P.R. (2000). 'Adult romantic attachments: theoretical developments, emerging controversies and unanswered questions.' *Review of General Psychology* 4: 132–54.

Hazen, C. and Shaver, P. (1987). 'Romantic love conceptualised as an attachment process.' *Journal of Personality and Social Psychology* 52: 511–24.

McGhie, A. (1979). *Psychology as Applied in Nursing*, 7th edn. Edinburgh: Churchill Livingston.

Nichols, K.A. (1993). *Psychological Care in Physical Illness*. London: Chapman and Hall.

Pencheon, D. and Koh, Y.M. (2000). 'Leadership and motivation (Career focus).' *British Medical Journal (Classified)* **321** (7256): 2.

Terry, P. (1997). *Working with the Elderly and Their Carers: a Psychodynamic Approach*. Hampshire: Palgrave McMillan.

Commentary on 'Visiting times'
Mary Paget

Unlike the chapters written by Lois and Sally (Chapters 5 and 7) which are both examples of strikingly unusual events in clinical practice, Mary's chapter reflects a situation that is not at all uncommon. Older patients are admitted to the hospital environment all the time. The majority of those will feel distressed and vulnerable and in many cases, members of their family will politely request that they be allowed to stay with them.

Mary describes one of the key people in her chapter, Mrs Jones, as being very distressed on her initial admission to the hospital ward. She may have felt a very realistic sense of panic and concern about her immediate future, worrying that she herself might die soon. We know that she was a widow; therefore her relationship with her husband had ended through death. She may also have 'lost' close friends through death or through being too unwell to pursue the relationships. In addition, Mrs Jones would have had little preparation for this admission as she was admitted as an emergency patient.

Terry (1997) uses the phrase 'persecuted by her losses' to describe a woman who, in common with many older people, had lost many important things from her life (Terry, 1997, p.122). It is easy to imagine that Mrs Jones may well have felt a sense of despair, disorientation and even disintegration. Mrs Jones' response to these feelings was to call out aloud for her daughter and to tell the nurses to leave her alone. Mary helpfully links this to the observations made by Robertson (1953) of small children when left behind by their mothers in hospital. The child protests at the separation in the only way they can, by crying and demonstrating anger. Mrs Jones' response to being separated from her main caregiver, her daughter, was similar. She called aloud for her daughter and in protest would not let the nurses attend to her.

However, after a few days, Mrs Jones became quieter, calling less often. Here too, there are comparisons with Robertson's children, when after a period of protest, the child becomes quieter and actual physical movement is reduced; indeed the child appears withdrawn and sad. This was perceived by the nurses as an improvement in Mrs Jones' condition. It may have been, but it could also be interpreted as the realisation that her daughter would not come and the recognition that calling aloud was pointless. It is possible then that her increasing quietness did not really signify adaptation, rather a depressed 'giving up'.

This analogy with childhood is not meant to infantilise the older patient, rather it invites us to consider that defences and coping strategies set up during childhood are embedded in all of us and are often utilised in later life, in times of stress. These strategies may even be accentuated in old age. Certainly, attachment figures are important at all ages, as was also demonstrated in Chapter 5. They are particularly needed for support and protection during times of uncertainty or illness.

When a relative is in hospital, nursing staff often encourage carers to claim back some time for themselves or to catch up on some much needed rest. However, as Mary points out, this may be impossible to achieve. The admission of a dependent patient to hospital often leaves the carer with unaccustomed time on their hands, time in which anxieties can multiply. The carer is caught in a waiting situation, and the uncertainty of the prognosis or long-term outcome may dominate their thinking. Such uncertainty is difficult to bear.

Mary considers why Mrs Jones' daughter felt the need to remain with her mother during the stay in hospital, suggesting that this may be related to a fear of her mother's further deterioration and possible transition to institutional care, or even concern about impending death. Like her mother, these realisations may have made Mrs Evans recognise a new external reality and the need to rethink their situation and modify her internal world. This, alongside the fear of a permanent loss, may have aroused in her additional emotions, from a sense of feeling not good enough to provide the necessary care for her mother, to a sense of relief that the burden of caring may soon be over, as well as the associated guilt that these feelings are likely to bring. Being together at this difficult time is likely to have provided them both with the psychological support that they needed.

Older people often express a fear of being institutionalised and forgotten by their families. For the carer, spending time at the bedside may be a way to convey that the older person is not forgotten, rather that their wellbeing remains central to the activities of their carer, as well as being a way to reciprocate the love and support given by the older person over the years.

It is worth considering whether Emma, the nurse, was also in a position that had left her feeling vulnerable. She too was in a new situation, as Mary had recently been appointed as her manager and was in the office at the time of the telephone call. For Emma, this may have given rise to a sense of uncertainty; what is this new manager going to be like? To what extent would Mary become involved in the day-to-day running of the ward concerned? When someone is appointed to a new role, there is always a period of readjustment within the working relationship, during which the individuals concerned are taking the measure of each other.

In this context, it is possible that Emma was still uncertain of Mary's management style and the extent to which boundaries would be enforced. Hospitals are places which are organised by rules, policies and protocols, with sometimes severe personal sanctions when rules are broken. Emma may have felt a sense of insecurity about 'breaking the rules' regarding visiting hours with her new manager present, deeming it safer to follow the rules. Mary, in her gentle response implicitly suggested that it was acceptable to 'break the rules' in this circumstance. It may also have signified to Emma that Mary would support her if she should use her discretion regarding the enforcement of some hospital rules.

Mary suggests that she has had a similar personal experience with an aged relative in hospital; indeed everyone has a range of life experiences which are brought into the work of nursing, all of which can influence and shape perceptions. Mary's own experiences clearly shaped her attitude in this particular situation, which she was keen to impart to Emma, but without compelling Emma to conform to her wishes. The desire to change Emma's mind, without undermining Emma's authority and confidence made the situation complicated. This interaction between colleagues suggests that the role of the manager in nursing is an area of complexity that is perhaps under-estimated.

It is also worth examining why Emma may not have desired visitors on the ward outside of visiting hours. There are always concerns about matters of confidentiality on an open hospital ward and there is also the belief that visitors 'clutter up the ward' and create extra work for nurses. It may be, however, that carers can relieve the nurses of responsibility for a range of tasks, such as helping people eat or taking them to the toilet. Perhaps nurses find it difficult to hand over care-giving activity or even find the scrutiny of an informal care-giver threatening. Certainly, it is harder to postpone activity with a patient, when a care-giver is present, keeping a watchful eye on events. Menzies Lyth (1988) recognised that nurses working within institutions adopt a range of defensive strategies and it is possible that these excuses are examples of such mechanisms in action.

References

Menzies Lyth, I. (1988). *Containing Anxiety in Institutions; Selected Essays*. Vol 1. London: Free Association Books.

Robertson, J. (1953). 'Some responses of young children to loss of maternal care.' Nursing Care **49**: 382–6.

Terry, P. (1997). *Working with the Elderly and their Carers. A Psychodynamic Approach.* Hampshire: Palgrave Macmillan.

Chapter 7
The bubble bath
Sally Williams

Introduction

This chapter aims to describe an incident from my paediatric nursing practice, and use several interpretations of psychodynamic frameworks to understand the incident and reveal a deeper meaning. This process will allow some of the unconscious dimensions within interpersonal relationships to be more clearly identified. This will aid understanding of the intensely complex emotions and feelings experienced during our day-to-day practice.

The incident

As an experienced paediatric nurse, I once had the fortunate opportunity to care for a ten-month-old child, whom I shall name 'James'. He had a complex medical condition, which was deteriorating. He had been a regular in-patient on the ward and at the time I cared for him, was suffering with acute liver failure. He had developed gross oedema, which made him both uncomfortable and miserable most of the time.

The shift was unusually quiet, on what was a busy paediatric ward. When I was in charge of the ward, I tried not to overburden myself with patients needing a lot of time-intensive care. I found it difficult to provide the time to care for children who need a lot of hands-on care, while managing the ward area, doctors' rounds and general enquiries. I would, therefore, allocate less of a patient workload to myself, in order to manage the ward area more effectively. However, the ward was quieter on this particular occasion and I decided to look after James myself.

Nurses and their patients

I can recall feeling a vague sense of unease, or apprehension, as I approached his cubicle. James at this time had complex care regimes, was technologically dependent and was difficult to physically move, without the fear of further compromising his general condition and adding to the discomfort he was experiencing. I am a confident, experienced practitioner but was unfamiliar with his routine. I was aware that this concerned me. As I approached the cot, a pair of glistening, sky blue eyes met me. They were accentuated by the discoloured yellow sclera commonly associated with liver failure, but they looked at me with a sense of mischief. Being unfamiliar with his routine suddenly didn't seem to be important any more. James smiled; he invited me to play with him.

We played that morning with an intensity that delighted us both. I gave him a luxurious bubble bath, which made him giggle so much, that people passing the room stopped to find out what all the noise was about. We played 'Boo', tickles and toys, and I can honestly admit I enjoyed playing that morning as much as he appeared to. When I became distracted he made even more noise, as if to remind me of his presence. When James tired and eventually drifted off to sleep, I carried him back to his cot and re-attached his various monitors, drips and feeds. He was exhausted and I felt exhilarated, both emotionally and spiritually. We had crossed the normal patient–nurse boundaries and had both experienced something more. We had both given something extra to the relationship and as a result, gained something very special from it.

I didn't care for James again because on my return to work, after my days off, I found he had deteriorated and had died. I felt as though he had chosen to share something very special with me. I have since moved on from nursing and commenced work as a nurse tutor, but this clinical experience is still as vivid now, as if it was yesterday. It feels significant to me, on both a personal and professional level.

Psychodynamics at work

Psychodyna-mics at work

The Oxford Dictionary (1995) defines 'psychodynamics' as 'the study of the activity of and the interrelation between the various parts of an individual's personality or psyche' (p. 1105). The study of psychodynamics taught me a different way of viewing my world, and the relationships I experienced through my day-to-day nursing care of children and families. This was a revelation. Studying psychodynamic theory gave me the opportunity to explore, in depth, and with a sense of honesty, what had helped me to engage with this particular patient.

As part of an MSc in Nursing, I had been exposed to several theories, which may help increase understanding of aspects of what are fundamental mental processes, used by nurses in our everyday activities when caring for patients. Such theories have been intriguing and have helped me gain the privilege of truly powerful insight into practice. Yet, this has also led me to question my own seemingly conscious, semi-conscious and possibly unconscious motivations, while delivering nursing care. While gaining this ultimate feeling of empowerment and emancipation with regard to my practice, the questioning and deliberations have been highly emotional, and thought provoking.

Paediatric nursing places an increased emphasis on developing fairly strong attachments to children, and their families in our care. While I believe that primitive maternal and paternal instincts are being provoked by exposure to sick, often distressed, crying infants, I have never allowed myself to question how this affects us as nurses, thereby influencing our ability to care for this client group. The experience with James described above is, for me, the essence of what it is to become really attached to a child in our care, to step beyond the socially and emotionally constructed boundaries, and 'engage' with another person.

This experience with James led me to examine the factors involved which allowed such a strong emotional bond to occur. What made me form an attachment with this child, at this time? What happened? Why does James feel so significant to me now? Can my actions and emotions be thought of as true 'attachment behaviour', or is it perhaps more appropriate to consider them as 'caretaking behaviour' (Bowlby, 1969).

Bowlby (1969) suggests that affectional bonding is built deep into our biological inheritance. In this paper he identifies how many forms of psychiatric disorders can be attributed to malfunctioning relationships experienced during childhood. This, he suggests, affects a person's capacity to make and maintain affectional bonds with significant others during adulthood. So critical is this ability to bond, that when a person's capacity to do so is compromised, it can result in a serious psychiatric disorder (Bowlby, 1969). This would suggest that bonding, or forming attachments to others, is a mutually beneficial activity, which protects us from potential psychological disorders. It is the core of our emotional well-being.

Ainsworth (1969) defines 'attachment' as:

> ... an affectional tie that one person (or animal) forms to another specific individual. Attachment is thus discriminating and specific ... attachments occur at all ages and do not necessarily imply immaturity or helplessness. To be sure the first tie is most likely to be formed with the mother, but this may soon be supplemented by attachments to a handful of other specific persons. (Ainsworth, 1969, p. 2)

The importance of such affectional bonds, or attachments, is also confirmed by other authors such as Gomez (1997). She suggests that we are born with in-built patterns of behaviour, which promote and maintain relationships. She goes further to suggest that this creating and maintaining of relationships can be thought of as essential to human development. This again supports the idea that the ability to form affectional bonds is a critical element of what it is to be human.

Within a care setting, nurses may be seen as ideally placed to initiate such bonds and attachments with their patients. The nurse is a frontline professional, prominent in most patients' care, and has to interact with the patient in order to deliver care. Thus, attachment work could be used as a core nursing skill to attend to the psychological needs of the patient. However, from personal experience of nursing, such bonding can be limited. Restrictions in resources, time, staff and just the sheer volume of work, make forming meaningful attachments with patients difficult.

What then is the patient's experience of being cared for, if the carer is detached? Can nursing care be delivered on a truly superficial level? The answer is 'yes', and I would go one step further to suggest that the vast majority of care is delivered with this detachment. Anna Dartington (1993) suggests '... attachment and its attendant emotionality is felt as such a threat to the system' (Dartington, 1993, p. 35). She refers to the hospital culture as not encouraging nurses to explore their emotional experiences. Indeed, she goes further, claiming attachment within the hospital system could be viewed as potentially overwhelming the nursing staff, thus affecting their clinical competence.

Does such intense, close, physical care lose anything if the person delivering it isn't bonding with the patient? Is it possible to deal with another person's suffering and pain without feeling at least some element of what Bowlby (1969) alludes to as our biological inheritance? In essence, can we play mother without feeling maternal?

Menzies Lyth (1988) explains the detachment within nursing as a 'defence' mechanism against anxiety, inherent in nurses, nursing and the hospital setting. She concludes that the social defence system within the hospital institution relies on primitive psychic defence mechanisms, facilitating the 'evasion' of anxiety. Therefore, in order to avoid anxiety, nurses avoid attachment, thereby preventing nursing care and practices which might allow development of full person-to-person relationships (Menzies Lyth, 1988). She does, however, recognise that the nursing profession's pursuit of avoiding anxiety through various strategies, results in anxiety and staff stress, which inevitably leads to adverse effects on patient recovery rates. Recommending alternative care practices, she heralds a need for the profession to embrace the emotional complexity of dealing with illness and suffering in patients, by containing nurses' anxiety and facilitating responses which use alternative defence mechanisms (see Chapter 4). So, while it is evident that we can nurse without being attached to our patients, this may prove detrimental to our patients' progress and our own psychological well-being.

My play experience with James felt as if I had experienced something more than just the delivery of care during the clinical shift. In this instance, I think I formed a deeper attachment with James. We bonded. The critical element provoking attachment and a caretaker response that morning was the mutuality of the pleasure of play. Children's communication is often through the medium of play. The process of play enabled me to form an attachment and caretaker relationship with James. It caused him to be interested in me and he was then able to hold my interest by involving me in his play.

The first mimic of a smile is made much of by parents, not so much because it is a primary social greeting, but as a breakthrough in communication. This is the first relationship that a child has and it is characterised by a cycle of reciprocity. The baby smiles and the parents smile back. This is referred to as an adaptive process which leads to a series of mutually satisfying behaviours. Based on the signals that the baby emits, the parents adapt their behaviour in order to incite a positive response from the infant (Goulet *et al.*, 1998). James held my attention by engaging me with a wide smile which made his face shine and his eyes twinkle.

Bowlby (1969) addresses the intensity of emotion, which affectional bonds can entail. He suggests the formation, maintenance, disruption and renewal of affectional bonds gives rise to very strong emotions. This was relevant to my time spent with James. In order to care for this child, and form an attachment to him, this required personal emotional investment. I felt for him; I empathised with his desire to play at that very difficult end-stage of his illness. I felt he needed me to assist him express himself as a child, not just a chronic condition.

For me, as a nurse and as a mother, to watch this child's determination to be 'alive' and express this in such an enlightening way was emotionally very significant. I felt exhilarated by his laughter, warmed by his gaze and yet deeply saddened and distressed by his predicament. This emotional intensity persisted, despite the fact that the encounter was fleeting in my life experience, especially when compared with other significant relationships I have had, most of which have spanned years. Therefore, this leads me to believe that some very significant encounters, which have a major impact on us, are brief. Maybe it is the very impact a person can have in such a short period of time that leaves us in awe of the intensity of emotions triggered.

It is suggested that it is part of our duty of care to consider the psychological well-being of our patients as well as their physical well-being (Casey, 1988). In order to empathise with our patients, there also develops an expectation for us to invest emotionally in our patients. In Bowlby's (1969) discussion of the reasons and causes for affectional bonds, he refers to the work of Anna Freud (1948) in developing the theory of what she terms 'cupboard love'. Freud (1948) suggests that a baby becomes attached to a mother out of material satisfaction, gained through infant feeding. Food, sex and dependency needs are highlighted as primary and secondary motivators for the acquisition of attachment figures and bonding by Bowlby (1969). He suggests that 'fear' is what motivates attachments as 'Protection from predators seems, therefore, more than likely to be the function performed by attachment behaviour, both in man and in other species'(Bowlby, 1969, p. 324). This is a very functional view of attachment, one not necessarily shared by all writers on the subject.

Ainsworth (2005) describes an affectional bond as a characteristic of the individual, and suggests that females, through evolutionary adaptation, are genetically biased to be both attachment orientated and more predisposed towards care-giving than males. Citing the female's need for greater protection when she has young, Ainsworth demonstrates how this may lead to greater attachment for security and comfort. Ainsworth (2005) concludes that affectional bonds have certain criteria, the maintenance of proximity, distress upon separation, joy upon reunion and grief at loss. The person with whom an affectional bond is formed becomes interchangeable with none other; they are unique to the person concerned. Ainsworth (2005) feels that this is the first bond formed by infants, usually to their mother as caregiver, and this attachment provides a secure base, which allows individual fulfilment in all of life's activities.

James can be described as being totally dependent in terms of basic care. Without others, he would not have his basic needs for food, warmth and comfort fulfilled. However, I believe he needed something more than this. I felt he was looking to me for some form of comfort and protection. Whether this was solely to provide physical protection, or emotional comfort I cannot be sure. Did he view me as someone who could protect him from his pain and discomfort by distracting him, or did he need emotional support in the form of a substitute maternal figure? I believe it is very hard in paediatric nursing not to consider yourself as to some degree a maternal figure. The desire to care for the baby in my arms provoked memories of what it was like to hold my own children. Knowing my children's dependence upon me when infants accentuates this automatic feeling of needing to care for babies in my professional role. This is what is referred to in psychodynamic theories as transference.

Nurses and their patients

Transference has been described in the literature as:

> ... the range of feelings, conflicts, defences and expectations of relationships projected unconsciously into a current relationship ... but originating in other, mostly earlier, relationships. (Hughes and Pengelly, 1997, p. 80)

O'Kelly (1998) suggests there is evidence of transference in almost all relationships. Dartington (1993) identifies the potential for the nurse to be seen as a mother figure, eliciting such emotional responses in patients because the nurse is seen as being a powerful expert, with the patient assuming a position of dependency and powerlessness. The response to a patient's transferred feelings is defined in the literature as 'counter-transference', which '...describes the reaction set off in the worker as a result of being receptive to the client's transferred feelings' (Salzberger-Wittenberg, 1970, p.18).

Such ideas would seem to support my initial feeling that there was some degree of transference in this interaction with James. The child provoked emotions within me, which I had experienced as a parent. The same feelings, of projected dependency and need, instigated caretaking responses within me, enabling me to care for James. I might have been feeling the unconscious desire to protect this child, as I have felt with my own children. That is, to protect him from the hospitalisation process, illness and suffering, and even from myself as a healthcare professional whose role and responsibilities can conflict with a maternal instinct to protect children from painful and unpleasant procedures.

It is customary to think of the patient's transference to the nurse and the nurse's counter-transference to the patient in relation to this transference (see Chapter 4). However, I may also have displaced the feelings I have for my own son, seemingly unconsciously towards James. The experience was emotionally a very positive one. It could be that the transference on this occasion highlighted the positive emotional aspects of what it is like to relate to, and care for, a small infant: something I could easily identify with. Thus the expectation was of a positive experience because I felt that James initiated some sort of bond. He played the part of an infant who wanted to engage me through his desire to play with me. This, perhaps, reminded me subconsciously of the positive emotions which I feel for my own children when they engage me in any form of play. This can be considered a core social skill associated with communicating with children and getting to know one another.

I doubt if my reaction to James would have been the same if he had cried and been irritable. I would probably have found myself attributing to him the more negative emotions which I associate with young infants. Thus my experience of his transference would have altered, affecting my counter-transference. The negativity, which may have arisen from memories of dealing with my own very difficult, colicky child, might have prevented the development of such a close bond with James. It was almost a collaborative relationship between James and me, within which we both had responsibility for playing a part. James' transference provoked my positive maternal feelings. He reflected the counter-transference of my maternal behaviour by assuming the role of the engaging infant.

Bowlby's (1969) attachment behaviour theory is understood by Ainsworth (1969) as 'interactional'. She suggests that his interpretation of a person is to be viewed in a social context, with their attachment behaviours 'interlocking with reciprocal behaviours of others; those of the infant are in inevitable interaction with the reciprocal behaviours of the mother figure' (Ainsworth, 1969, p. 34). The reciprocity of the experience I shared with James was fundamental to the relationship. Without this engagement, I doubt whether the emotions and feeling would have been as strong.

The child's ability to reveal their emotions in a less guarded way than perhaps an adult means they tend to be far easier to read emotionally. James, presumably, responded to me in the same way he would to his mother. He would possibly associate the uniform I was wearing with food and attention. If he can engage me, then he will probably gain more from the relationship in terms of, perhaps, attention. We were both experiencing feelings associated with maternal attachment, which has elements of reciprocity and reliance, which inevitably initiates a caretaking response from another who has the ability to provide for us.

Another of Bowlby's (1969) theories describes care given between a mother and child as a process, which he calls 'caretaking'. He concludes that this exists as complementary behaviour to attachment behaviour. It is described in the paper, most notably in the relationship that exists between a mother and her young, although it can be displayed by fathers, and any other dominant animal towards their young or any subordinate of his group. The emphasis within Bowlby's (1969) work is on the attachment behaviour rather than this 'caretaking', which is considered as complementary. 'Caretaking' however, could be regarded as critical to the survival of the species. If the infant cannot generate such a response in a parent, which would make them wish to care for this child and nurture it, then the child would not be able to survive. Without the ability to attract a parent or primary care-giver who wants to care for the infant, their survival is ultimately jeopardised. They are reliant on the 'caretaking' of the parent, with whom they will then form an attachment. The parent may well feel emotionally attached to the infant, but unless they act as the child's caretaker, the child will not survive. Ainsworth (2005) draws attention to the importance of the strength of the emotional bond between parent and child, suggesting that the quality of care-giving is directly related to the bond formed between the two. So the concept of 'caretaking' becomes critical to a child's ability to survive and thus a prerequisite in forming emotional attachments to the parent.

It could be seen as part of my job, and so my professional responsibility, to provide such caretaking for the children whom I nurse. Indeed I consider my professional caretaking to be critical to the survival of a sick infant. This relationship, however, is further enhanced if, as in the case of James, I form an emotional attachment to the child. My caretaking was critical to his survival and yet by becoming emotionally attached to him, we experienced far more than basic caretaking. Therefore the child and I benefited, not just physically from the good quality of undisturbed care that I was able to deliver that morning, but also emotionally, as we both gained something from the experience. This was important not just for James and what he was able to experience and enjoy, but also it had importance in my mind for the way I perceived his emotional needs that morning. I was able to deliver that extra level of care, which is so often sacrificed, due to the other pressures of work on the ward.

For me, personally, as a professional nurse, there is a difference between 'giving care' to a patient and 'caring for' a patient. The first requires some delivery of basic nursing interventions, in much the same way as Bowlby (1969) refers to a parent 'caretaking' a child, supplying what is needed to another person to ensure their needs are met. Washing, feeding and giving medicine are examples of this type of nursing input, whilst 'caring' for a patient suggests an emotional investment on the part of the nurse. This is what Bowlby (1969) refers to as becoming 'emotionally attached', in this instance becoming emotionally attached to the patient when delivering care, which will facilitate a more empathic, holistic, approach to the child and family where necessary.

The emphasis now on target driven healthcare systems, which need to be able to demonstrate their effectiveness and outcomes in clearly defined health gains for the patient is, for me, problematic. It is difficult, if not impossible, to quantify or measure the difference between 'giving care' and 'caring' for the patient. The difficulty in quantifying, and so proving the value of emotional investment in patient care, is frustrating. To suggest that it 'feels better' or emotionally is 'more rewarding' to care for your patient at this more involved level, appears impossible to sell to a financially driven, medicalised, healthcare environment, where the emphasis is on 'curing' and not 'caring'.

Significance

Significance

From my own perspective, the work with James is more significant to me because of personal changes, which occurred in my life at that time. It included the transition from being a practising paediatric nurse to that of a nurse tutor. This has, on the surface, been fairly uneventful; however I have felt at times a degree of uncertainty about my future career and have regarded the transition with a slight sense of loss. This again has aspects which are echoed in Bowlby's (1969) attachment theory. The framework can be extended to include the loss of attachment to something such as a clinical nursing career. Much of what I experienced as a paediatric nurse led me to form close emotional attachments, not only to the children I cared for, but also to the families and colleagues I worked with over a prolonged period of time.

There is a sense of loss that I may never again be an expert nurse within that field. I have lost part of my professional and personal identity. There is a definite sense of loss when I stop to consider some of the close relationships I have had with children whom I nursed, first as babies, then toddlers and then on into school years. I feel as though I have almost emotionally abandoned some of the families I have cared for over the years. That I feel such a sense of loss indicates that I must have been emotionally attached to them, at some level of emotional consciousness. Bowlby (1969) refers to this process and suggests that actual loss of affectional bonds gives rise to feelings of sorrow. To some extent I have lost something very precious in being denied the close contact with my patients, but I have also lost my identity which was defined by those same, close, working relationships with children and their families. The incident for me was one of the last, intensive nursing experiences which occurred before I changed my job. It signifies what I feel I did best for my patients: deliver expert care with an empathic and holistic approach, which could be mutually rewarding.

Bowlby's framework

Bowlby's framework

Whilst the revelations Bowlby made in the 1950s and 1960s regarding attachment theory are useful in understanding this practice exemplar, there are details which differ from his theoretical framework concerning the time it takes to develop such emotional bonds within relationships. The literature from Bowlby's work identifies attachment as being developed over a period of time. This is also emphasised in the paper by Ainsworth (1969) who describes 'attachment' as '... not a term to be applied to any transient relation or to a purely situational dependency transaction' (Ainsworth, 1969, p. 2).

I do not believe that what I delivered to James in that instance was 'a purely situational dependency transaction', where 'what is sought and received' (Ainsworth, 1969, p. 2) is of utmost significance. I believe there was a degree of attachment experienced within the relationship, there was limited longevity, but the content was no less important. Whether James displayed attachment behaviour towards me specifically, or whether it would be more realistic to suggest that he, through repeated long admissions to hospital, was becoming attached to the understanding that the 'uniform' I wore represented food, attention and familiarity, I do not know; it cannot be proven because of his age and cognitive level. However, what is clear to me now is that I was engaged in some sort of emotional bond with James, quite likely as a result of my counter-transference of maternal feelings towards him.

I have concluded, through using the frameworks and theories of Bowlby (1969) and Ainsworth (1969), that as part of my role as a nurse, I formed frequent, often transient, relationships with parents and children, at what can be considered a stressful, critical point in their lives. It might be suggested that I was, and still am really, emotionally attached to the essence of these relationships, which for me symbolises good nursing care. It is perhaps an emotional attachment to the profession of nursing that is best understood through my affectional bonds to those for whom I cared. This, therefore, is why I feel that the incident with James is so significant for me now at a time when I am searching for a new attachment, affectional bond, with my new experiences as a nurse tutor.

Conclusion

It can be seen that by using a psychoanalytic framework, the experience of nursing practice can be better understood, and the emotional relationships which entwine everyday nursing care and delivery can be most usefully examined. Through using the work on attachment theory and affectional bonds by Bowlby (1969) and Ainsworth (1969, 2005) I can appreciate the more complex aspects of a clinical experience, and use that interpretation to share an increased understanding with others, within a nursing context. The ultimate aim, however, must be to increase our understanding of the complexities of 'caring' for patients and their families, in an attempt to improve our ability to deliver nursing 'care' in the future.

References

Ainsworth, M.D.S. (1969). 'Object relations, dependency, and attachment: a theoretical review of the infant-mother relationship.' *Child Development* **40**: 969–1025.

Ainsworth, M.D.S. (2005). 'Attachments and other affectional bonds across the life cycle.' In *Attachment Across the Life Cycle*, eds. C.M. Parkes, J. Stevenson-Hind and P. Marris. London: Tavistock, Routledge, pp. 33–51.

Bowlby, J. (1969). 'Affectional bonds: their nature and origin.' In *Progress in Mental Health: Proceedings of the Seventh International Congress on Mental Health*, ed. H. Freeman. London: J. and A. Churchill, pp.319–27.

Casey, A. (1988). 'A partnership with child and family.' *Senior Nurse* **8**(4): 8–9.

Dartington, A. (1993). 'Where angels fear to tread. Idealism, despondency, and inhibition in thought in hospital nursing.' *Winnicott Studies* **7** (Spring): 21–41.

Freud, A. (1948). 'The psychoanalytic study of infantile feeding disturbances.' *Psychoanalytic Study of the Child* **2**: 119–32.

Gomez, L. (1997). 'John Bowlby: Attachment theory.' In *An Introduction to Object Relations*. London: Free Association Books.

Goulet, C., Bell, L., St-Cyr, D., Paul, D. and Lang, A. (1998). 'A concept analysis of the parent-infant relationship.' *Journal of Advanced Nursing* **28** (5): 1071--81.

Hughes, L. and Pengelly, P. (1997). *Staff Supervision in a Turbulent Environment*. London: Jessica Kingsley.

O'Kelly, G. (1998). 'Countertransference in the nurse patient relationship: a review of the literature.' *Journal of Advanced Nursing* **28**(2): 391–7

Menzies Lyth, I. (1988). 'The functioning of social systems as a defence against anxiety.' In *Containing Anxiety in Institutions: Selected Essays*, Vol. 1. London: Free Association Books.

Salzberger-Wittenberg, I. (1970). 'Transference and countertransference.' In *Psycho-analytic Insight and Relationships: A Kleinian Approach*. London: Routledge.

The Concise Oxford Dictionary. (1995) 9th edn. Oxford: Clarendon Press. p. 1105

Commentary on 'The bubble bath'
Mary Paget

In the preceding chapter, Sally writes a heart-warming account of a morning spent with a dying infant of ten months of age. In this account, Sally clearly demonstrates attunement to the needs of the infant (James) on that particular morning and a quality of care-giving that most nurses aspire to. There is one particularly unusual aspect to the relationship that developed between Sally and James that morning and that is the readiness with which James both invited attention and responded to it. Unusual, because most infants demonstrate some reluctance to bond with strangers in the way that James did. And Sally was indeed a stranger as they had never met before that morning. It is striking that he was so comfortable with Sally. One wonders why?

Weinfield *et al.* (1999) suggest that the need to form attachments is an integral part of the human personality, but where there is no continuous or stable presence, such as in some forms of institutional care, children may remain unattached or have difficulty establishing an attachment relationship. Within the orphanage setting, the needs of infants can be met inconsistently by any number of providers, in a routine, non-individual manner, giving the infant little opportunity to develop trust with a preferred attachment figure (Chesney, 2008). Roy, Rutter and Pickles (2004) suggest that up to a fifth of institutionalised children lack a selective attachment relationship. However, the hospital setting differs somewhat from other forms of institutional care. In the modern hospital, parents are encouraged to be with their offspring for the duration of the child's stay, but where other siblings exist, this may not be possible and the infant may spend long periods of time, like James, without a primary caregiver's presence. Was it the case that James' quick attachment to Sally was the consequence of indiscriminate attachment, in turn a result of his long periods of institutional care in hospital? One feels reluctant to conclude this in the face of the intensity and mutual satisfaction of the relationship described.

Fonagy (2001) contends that the physical absence of the mother figure is not the key to understanding the infant's response in this sort of situation. Rather, it is the infant's own appraisal or evaluation of the mother's departure, in the context of her expected behaviour. This suggests that the anxieties occasioned by separation from the mother are moderated by a complex set of (unconscious) evaluative processes, even in small infants. In these circumstances, what the infant expects relates directly to what has been experienced before. Sroufe and Waters (1977) liken this to a sense of 'felt security' rather than the mere regulation of physical distance and suggest that this sense is influenced by mood, illness or even fantasy.

Nurses and their patients

On this day, James seemed to have no difficulty in establishing a relationship with Sally. As Sally describes it, 'I think I formed a deeper attachment with James. We bonded.' This tends to suggest that something more may have been happening than is explained by the various theories, or that James' anxieties had been so well managed in his short life that he felt secure, even in the absence of his mother.

Something important, that we may never fully understand, was going on in his mind to enable the contact he and Sally had. One also has to note the power of it, how James unconsciously made himself unforgettable in Sally's mind. Knowing as we do that he later died, this seems humbling and profound.

Sally discusses the idea of transference within this relationship, suggesting that James' need and desire to play was projected into Sally, who responded in kind. As a mother already, Sally recognised this need and responded as a mother would with her own child. This reciprocity of activity led to the beginnings of an attachment which was then strengthened through the play experience, with a lasting effect on Sally's emotions. Certainly, this emotional link led to a quality of care-giving over and above the usual level.

An emphasis on the quality of care-giving prevails in psychodynamic theory. Winnicott (1988) in particular, refers to the need for the mother-figure to effectively handle the infant's anxieties and impulses and to adapt themselves to the needs of the infant. He suggests that mothers develop an 'amazing capacity' to identify with their infants which makes them 'able to meet the basic needs of the infant in a way that no machine can imitate and no teaching can reach' (Winnicott, 1988, pp. 36–7). This capacity requires time to develop and involves adaptations that match the infant's changing needs. According to Winnicott, this skilled handling of the infant's physical and emotional needs allows the infant to remain integrated, to remain together and not to fall victim to its own anxieties and panic. The mother that is able to achieve this is considered to be 'good enough'. For such a relationship to develop there needs to be time as well as an emotional investment.

This contrasts strongly with the current face of health care which seems to be more about 'just enough' care rather than providing 'good enough' care. This may be partly a result of working in a target-driven service, in which the numbers cared for take precedence over the quality of that care. The personal desire

Commentary on 'The bubble bath'

to do good, to provide the best care for one's patients, conflicts directly with the institutional need to do just enough and may account for some of the stresses and anxieties felt by nurses when caring for patients.

Menzies Lyth (1988) and Skogstad (1997) suggested that contact with patients and relatives can generate severe anxieties and defences emerge to prevent the individual from becoming dysfunctional (see Chapters 1, 3 and 4). Such defences arise unconsciously and can be used very rigidly. The development of a 'hard shell' would be one illustration. A 'shell' allows the nurse to provide essential physical care rather than the level of care that demands any emotional investment. It was Menzies Lyth's contention that such rigid use of what she termed 'primitive defences' may impoverish both nurse and patient. She recommended that nurses needed help to face, rather than avoid the anxieties generated by the work, as this was the only way that they could be modified and reduced (Menzies Lyth,1988, p. 77).

On the morning that Sally describes, far from being defended, she seems to have been very open to her patients' emotional needs. The clinical area was relatively quiet, and instead of undertaking several tasks before moving on to another child, Sally was able to care for James in the most thorough way and in this time they 'clicked'. This suggests that in the right circumstances, the emotional components of care can be built up over a very short period of time, yet can linger for some years, as is evident from Sally's story. Is this emotional work of nursing created by the nature of the role and the requirements of patients? If so, then it needs recognition in the daily context of care, with sufficient time being provided to build effective relationships with patients.

In Sally's case, clinical supervision (see Chapters 13 and 14) could have helped her elicit a better understanding of the relationship that developed on that morning and why the events of that morning still remain vivid in her memory. I believe that Sally was indeed lucky to have had the opportunity to experience such intense feelings in caring for a patient, even if it was also very poignant, especially as it came towards the end of a stage in Sally's career. This opportunity to give excellent care, rather than 'just enough' care is something that nurses should, but cannot always, aspire to. But then maybe it takes a certain kind of nurse who has the capacity to see what is required, in the way that Sally did.

References

Chesney, M. (2008) 'Fostering the parent-child attachment relationship.' www.med.umn.edu/peds/iac/topics/attachment/home.html (Accessed 17 July 2008)

Fonagy, P. (2001) *Attachment Theory and Psychoanalysis*. New York: Other Press.

Menzies Lyth, I. (1988). *Containing Anxiety in Institutions: Selected Essays*, Vol. I. London: Free Association Books.

Roy, P., Rutter, M. and Pickles, A. (2004). 'Institutional care: associations between overactivity and lack of selectivity in social relationships.' *Journal of Child Psychology and Psychiatry and Allied Disciplines* 45(4): 866–73.

Skogstad, W. (1997). 'Working in a world of bodies: defensive techniques on a medical ward – a psychoanalytical observation.' *Psychoanalytic Psychotherapy* 11(3): 221–41.

Sroufe, L.A. and Waters, E. (1977). 'Attachment as an organisational construct.' *Child Development* 48: 1184–99.

Weinfield, N.S., Sroufe, L.A., Egeland, B. and Carlson, E.A. (1999). 'The nature of individual differences in infant-caregiver attachment.' In *Handbook of Attachment, Theory, Research and Clinical Applications*, eds. J. Cassidy and P.R. Shaver. New York: Guilford Press, pp. 68–88.

Winnicott, D. (1988). *Babies and their Mothers.* London: Free Association Books.

Chapter 8
Sadie's baby

Grace Sansom

Introduction

This chapter explores a complex nursing issue from the field of old age psychiatry. The account referred to is called 'Sadie's baby' and examines a series of occurrences experienced during one lady's stay at a long-term facility for people with dementia. Psychodynamic ideas are used to try to understand what happened.

The scenario

The scenario

I first met Sadie on a continuing care hospital ward, where I was the new night nursing manager. Sadie appeared as a large, white-haired, jolly old lady with wicked smiling eyes. She had a beautiful beaming face, with very few lines on her near perfect skin. She was sitting in a big wing-backed chair facing the door next to the fireplace, nursing, with a securely wrapped blanket around her body or 'Welsh fashion', a baby doll.

I could not fail to be attracted to her and what she was doing, and so I headed straight towards her, bent down and said 'hello'. The nursing staff introduced me to Sadie and then to her 'baby'. She beamed when I admired the doll and presented her to me for closer inspection. I commented on how pretty she was and asked her name, 'Baby' she said, 'Baby'. Her eyes were sparkling and full of pride, giving loving looks at the doll in the shawl. I left Sadie very content and proceeded to speak with the other ladies in the room. Later I asked the nursing staff to explain the significance of the doll to me.

They told me of the difficulties when Sadie first came into long-term care. How resistant she had been to any form of physical care, of which she required a considerable amount, as Sadie was immobile and doubly incontinent. As a large, physically strong lady, prone to aggressive outbursts, physical nursing interventions became times of distress for all involved. Early in her dementia, while being cared for by her doting late husband, Burt, she had begun to take great comfort from comforting one of her grandchildren's dolls, becoming quite loath to part with it. Sadie's daughter purchased a similar doll for her daughter, leaving Sadie with the original.

Although Burt did not complain about Sadie's behaviour, she was very difficult at times. With the arrival of 'baby', life became a little easier for him physically. Her preoccupation with the baby distracted her from the distress previously displayed at bath times, mealtimes, attending the toilet and dressing. All things seemed possible with 'baby' around and she remained in her own home until the sudden death of Burt.

Her daughter attempted to care for Sadie but the situation was fraught. Finally, events spiralled out of control when Sadie smacked her four-year-old granddaughter for being a 'naughty baby' and was admitted for long-term hospital care. The daughter suggested the doll be brought into hospital, but worried that hospital staff might disapprove. Indeed not all the ward nurses did approve of Sadie having this doll. Some staff felt it undermined her as an adult and some would even take it away, saying: 'She is not having that when I'm on duty!' Reports of aggressive behaviour would follow, leading to a distressed Sadie. This continuing situation troubled me and I spoke to the ward sister about the problem.

We then had a visit from a previously unseen son. He demanded that the 'silly doll' be taken from his mother and said: 'How dare you treat her as if she was in second childhood'. He told the ward sister it was degrading to see his mother like this and said he would report staff to the highest authority, should he see the doll again. The sister, although in disagreement with him could not stand up to him, and the doll was put away.

I was furious that night. The decision was wrong and proved detrimental to Sadie, who was very distressed, her mood was low and the sparkle in her eyes was gone. Supper-time was a nightmare, and undressing her for bed felt like an assault. We could not go on like this and searched for the doll, to no avail. Sadie did not sleep and required night sedation. The following morning this was reported with a request for reconsideration of the care plan. The next night the doll was found and given back to Sadie.

I knew I had to sort this problem out, so I swapped duties with the ward manager, knowing I would then meet this son. I did not have to wait long; he came in, Sadie had the doll, he was angry and I was scared. I asked him if he would step into my office so that we could discuss this issue. He shouted at me and asked who did I think I was, making his mother look 'simple and childlike' in front of all the others. I let him continue as he needed to get it out of his system, and he eventually ran out of steam.

I maintained my voice at a normal or quieter tone than usual and explained how long and in what circumstances I had nursed his mother. I explained that I fully understood his concerns, but professionally I had genuine reasons for believing the doll had a special significance for his mother. I explained to him the difference it made, especially from my own experiences at night. He listened intently and then said: 'Well, I'll go over your head. I want to see the consultant.' I then offered to arrange the appointment for him and this stopped him in his tracks. He just looked at me and said: 'You actually believe this doll helps her get through don't you?' 'Yes,' I replied, 'and so do many of my staff, but we also respect that you care enough about your mother to want to do the right thing by her.' 'Tell me more about the difference it makes,' he said. So I recounted little tales, of her stroking and cooing to the doll and sometimes how she would fall out with the doll, but generally how calm it made her. I asked if he could think why this might be and he began to go back to when he was a little boy and how she would tell him about the babies she had nursed and loved. He asked me if I thought she was withdrawing back to those days, remembering or believing she was a nanny again. I said I was not really sure, as none of us can know what another person is thinking, but it was possible. All I knew was that it made her happy and I had seen this occur. He got up to leave, so I asked: 'What about the consultant then, shall I arrange that?' He just replied: 'Let her keep the doll, you make sure she does.' 'Thank you,' I said, and he left.

It was then written in Sadie's care plan that she was to have 'baby' whenever she liked, making the staff very happy. Sadie appeared none the wiser that this confrontation had taken place.

Discussion

Discussion

Using psychodynamic ideas, this situation will be explored to elicit an understanding of how the fundamental processes of communication and interaction within the caring context are understood, prioritised and utilised. As 'baby' takes on such a vital function within this account, key players will be discussed in terms of their relationship with, and the effect of, 'baby' upon them. Relevant psychodynamic theory will be drawn upon to explore, understand, and critically analyse their perspectives.

Psychodynamic theory is concerned with ideas focusing on individual motives, conflicts, and imaginings, described as unconscious mental processes, due to the individual's lack of awareness of their existence (Kitwood, 1997). Psychodynamic theories are collectively about the study of the mind, which stresses active unconscious forces within the personality. They include ideas regarding the inner causes of behaviour which are associated with feelings, conflicts, instinctive drives, and various unconscious motivational factors (Gross, 1991).

During the time of my experience with Sadie, I admit to having given limited thought as to why 'baby' was so important. I accepted it was, but did not know why. The assumption made was that the doll reminded Sadie of happier times, to which she was now mentally withdrawing. As I explored various psychodynamic theories, I realised that I had not given these ideas any consideration. With hindsight, I think unconscious mental processes, rather than knowledge, were being drawn upon.

'Baby' and Sadie

In the described scenario 'baby', an inanimate doll, becomes almost as important as Sadie herself, in terms of its effect upon her and all the participants. An explanation for this may be found within the realms of the perceived strength of meaning attached to the doll. This appeared to symbolise some aspect of Sadie's life and the situation in which she now found herself. Exploration from a psychodynamic perspective may help reveal this.

Klein (1963) suggests, when considering behaviour from a psychoanalytical viewpoint, that it is necessary to scrutinise how individual personalities develop from infancy to maturity. Klein claims that the capacity to love and to sense persecution is deep rooted within the infant's earliest mental processes, focused primarily on the mother. It is from these roots that insight is gained into the way our mind, habits, and views are built from the primitive fantasies and emotions of childhood, to the most complex of adult displays. Klein suggests that the ego can develop strength, by the mother being taken into the inner world of the child as a good and dependable object, through the use of the defence mechanism of introjection. If the mother is loving, giving and helping towards the child, then her good aspects will be the first good object that the infant takes into his inner world. Erikson (1995) claims that what an infant learns through its interactions with its mother is a position of 'basic trust' versus 'basic mistrust' of the world and the people in it. Therefore, the first relationship is regarded as crucial for healthy development, acting as the prototype upon which future relationships are built and sustained.

Building on the internalised good object, the child can begin to accept and identify with others in a positive way, thus contributing to a stable personality. If however, persecutory anxiety overwhelms, then the ego (roughly speaking, the sense one has of one's self, of being a 'self') desires to 'split' loved objects from dangerous ones, in order to protect them. A battle can ensue within the mind of the baby and if he has enough experience of the good mother he will cling to this and feed, thrive, and preserve his belief in the good object and his capacity to love it. Survival may totally depend on him having established trust and love with the mother, for without this feeling, he may be exposed to a hostile world which he fears could destroy him and has the potential to do so.

Sadie may have internalised enough of the good mother to be able to search, even in times of unbelievable distress, for the good object inside her and possibly project this feeling on to the doll, unconsciously. She may well see herself as the doll, thereby preserving and restoring the good internal object she is in fear of losing, due to dementia. Sadie clutches the doll, which is wrapped up in a shawl for comfort. She may be trying to demonstrate the way she would like to be held, loved, and contained with clothes, in the shawl, but also, she may be conveying her memory of having been cared for in this way and her memories of her own good ability to provide this care as a mother/nanny herself.

Times of potential great distress were minimised by 'baby', especially with physical interventions such as bathing, which required removal of clothing. Being exposed can be very threatening for older people who may consider nudity as immoral, with clothing often seen as a protective barrier against society. Due to the cognitive decline of persons with dementia, a full appreciation of what is happening to them isn't always easily understood. Consequently, attempts to assist someone to wash or bathe, which involve removal of clothing, can become anxiety provoking which at best may be perceived as a personal attack, and at worst as a dreadful feeling of disintegration as if the skin is being removed with the clothing. Prior to 'baby', bath times were pretty dire for all involved, as the threat of clothing being removed without her fully understanding why, was very frightening for Sadie and she fought against this with all her might.

Winnicott's (1988, p. 31) ideas may be used to suggest that Sadie was drawing on instincts seen in infancy. These include 'aggressiveness in the live baby', due to a fear of falling apart. The baby displays this when in need of nourishment, being undressed, or unwrapped, as he screams, kicks, scratches and throws open his body. There may be a similarity here between the fears of total devastation in the baby and the bewilderment and utter terror that Sadie felt, to make her react in a similar way. She was merely acting on instinct, much like a baby. To ease such anxiety or when going to sleep, Winnicott (1958) suggests that babies commonly display many activities, for example, mouthing or sucking part of an object, plucking or caressing it, and accompanying these activities with babbling sounds. They can find comfort in objects such as a blanket, part of a blanket, a tune, or a mannerism. Sadie may have been using 'baby' in this way.

Winnicott (1958) referred to these activities as transitional phenomena, and going further, suggests that such activities may emerge as vitally important to the infant. The use of the doll in Sadie's situation might be explained as a 'transitional object' and a 'transitional phenomenon' (Winnicott, 1958). A transitional object is an object of great importance; he refers to it as the original 'Not-Me' possession. He suggested this period of transition was an intermediate time of experience between the infant sucking his thumb, that is, 'Me' and a teddy bear, that is, 'Not-me'. The good enough mother inevitably fails in a developmentally appropriate way, allowing the infant to believe he has some magical force that makes things happen and perpetuates this illusionary state, thus enabling the infant to deal with the looming reality of mother's separateness. By being absent from the baby for short periods, leaving the baby with another carer, or making the baby wait for gratification, the 'good enough' mother allows her infant to adapt mentally, understand, and therefore develop, whereas the overprotective mother responds on the spot and runs the risk of preventing the infant from developing the capacity to tolerate loss.

Winnicott (1958), while accepting the transitional object as symbolic of the mother, or some part of her such as the breast, notes it is not symbolism being displayed. Symbolism would be a time when the infant can actually distinguish between fantasy and fact, that is between 'me' and 'not-me'. The use of the transitional object is the journey the infant takes to get there. In Sadie's case, 'baby', as a transitional object, may have provided her with the means by which she could control something within her environment, as all around her is strange and anxiety provoking. The object allows her to believe she has control, not only over 'baby' but indeed over others, as they actually get caught up in the idea of this illusion. For instance, nursing staff responded positively to Sadie's 'baby' and rallied around to support her in the struggle to keep the doll, thus helping her to gain control over her situation.

In terms of Sadie, would Winnicott (1958) consider her 'baby' as a transitional object? Sadie assumed rights over the doll to love or reject, an alternative would not do. The doll seemed to be alive for Sadie, giving her pleasure when she stroked it and offered it to others for admiration. However, it was impossible to tell if Sadie really believed the doll was a baby or not. The importance of the doll was never forgotten, on the contrary the pleasure did not fade, her eyes continued to sparkle when 'baby' was introduced. However, Sadie's 'baby' only partially fulfils Winnicott's (1958) transitional object criteria, as of course here we are not dealing with a child, but an adult woman with dementia. Special qualities of the transitional object, as proposed by Winnicott, include the ability for the infant to move on and relegate the object to limbo; in Sadie's case this progression was unlikely to occur.

Gomez (1997) identifies that the young baby has the potential to be 'on the brink of unthinkable anxiety' if the baby is not attended to by a good enough mother (Gomez 1997, p. 88). The baby can easily fall into an agonising state, going to pieces, losing relations with the body, and the world, with no way of communicating his/her needs. Winnicott referred to this as the sensation of 'annihilation' with a potential for such horrors to return in later life, when anxieties are overwhelming. People suffering psychiatric illness often express feelings of 'falling apart', 'going to pieces', and more commonly, 'breaking down'. Winnicott (1988) suggests that this is not fear of an unknown situation but rather a return to a previous state of dereliction.

It is speculative but possible to suggest that, in Sadie's case, she used the doll as a transitional object to help her guard against the anxiety of an unbearable state of disintegration. Suffering from dementia had clouded her cognitive abilities, in terms of judgement and reasoning. The strange unknown situation in which she found herself seems to have provoked severe anxiety. Defending against this anxiety, by imaginatively returning to a more comforting time with mother may have been the best instinctual reaction she could invoke. With the introduction of the doll, her initial anxiety appeared to subside, only to reappear on its removal.

We can only guess at the significance the doll held for Sadie, as it is she who bestowed upon it its symbolic power. It is possible she was trying to restore the good object within herself that felt lost. The doll had the function of helping to soothe the suffering and losses she might have been feeling. She might have perceived her ability to reject the doll as the retention of some element of control over the strange situation in which she found herself, as she was able to love it, and reject it, without fear of reprisal.

Sadie had lost her husband, home, family, and independence. She also lost her caring role for babies, which was her purpose in life, and her rational ability, due to her illness. To deal with such separation and loss, she demonstrates coping, and containing, to the best of her ability, through the use of the doll. Through this, Sadie may be trying to reclaim the professional caring role familiar to her previous experience. By demonstrating that she is caring for the doll, it is possible for her to deny her own dependency. Conversely, she may be experiencing herself through the object, the doll, thus protecting herself from total exposure and disintegration. She might never be able to use the doll as a truly transitional object, as no transition, or journey forward in developmental terms would be taking place, but it may help her psychological survival in the present.

The fact that Sadie is an adult is not of importance to Gomez (1997) who claims that special objects in adulthood can be remnants of original feelings and attachments we held for our first carer, often mother. Bowlby (1969) suggests that the patterns on which adults model their affectional bonds are determined during childhood, often resulting from the first and foremost relationship with the mother. Attachment is classed as a distinct behaviour and whether this is displayed as crying, calling, following, or clinging, if it results in proximity to an attachment figure, then it is attachment behaviour. Bowlby (1969, p. 323) claims that attachment behaviour is not merely displayed by the young; on the contrary, he considers it as a 'normal and healthy part of human nature from the cradle to the grave'. Indeed, I have witnessed many adults bring a significant small object or toy into hospital with them.

Bretherton (1991) discusses historical development and current thinking regarding attachment theory. This area is rich, interesting, and totally applicable for consideration when caring for people with dementia. Rather than considering Sadie as regressing, in a negative manner, as many of us probably had in the clinical setting, Bowlby (1969) suggests that far from being regressive, attachment phenomena should be viewed as perfectly normal behaviour. He suggests that:

> In illness or emergency, each of us seeks the comforting presence of those we know and trust and, moreover, feels troubled, unhappy and anxious if for any reason they are not available. (Bowlby, 1969, p. 323)

Regression, an unconscious defence mechanism, is understood to be the retreat from a current anxiety, by reverting to less mature behaviour, once used to dispel anxiety and inner tension (see

Chapter 3). Nichols (1993) claims that illness and injury produce two outcomes: the experience of threat and the experience of loss, emotional reactions that can be harder to bear than the illness itself. It is possible that due to such loss, Sadie regressed. However, McGhie (1979) suggests that the regressive response has a tendency to be a transient reaction, with the individual returning to mature behaviour once the situation has resolved. With Sadie the situation did not resolve. I propose that what may have begun as regression was unable to resolve the internal anxiety and therefore a more permanent coping strategy was sought. This took the form of attachment phenomena, coupled with the opportunity to utilise the doll as a transitional object. I now consider Sadie to be displaying attachment behaviour, as opposed to regressive behaviour.

Bowlby (1969) suggests that attachment behaviour is most frequently summoned when individuals are less able to fend for themselves or when they are ill or handicapped. Miesen (1992) identifies feeling unsafe and insecure as common features of dementia, as strange situations become a permanent part of experience. The need for security and safety to deal with strange experiences can trigger attachment behaviour. The more danger perceived, the more attachment behaviour is displayed. Bowlby (1969) hypothesises that attachment behaviour, as a method of avoiding isolation by gaining proximity to a familiar object, is one way of avoiding separation anxiety. Attachment behaviour is foremost when we are separated from a person or object with which we have a strong affectional bond, in other words when we are unable to find our mother figure or her adult representative.

Miesen (1992) claims that a person with dementia is caught up in an experience comparable to bereavement and which can never be resolved. This becomes a vicious circle where dementia activates attachment behaviour, yet ensures that old or new attachments cannot be obtained. However, in Sadie's case, she appears to use the doll to enable her to form new attachments. The fact that she displayed such strong responses to the threat of its removal, alerting me to react to her plight and take on a caretaker role, is surely worthy of recognition. This demonstrates the strong sense of personhood and well-being that remained, even with advanced dementia where common forms of communication are hampered (Kitwood, 1997). The pure joy on

Sadie's face on rediscovering the doll even after a short time was enormous and worth all the problems that had to be overcome to make this happen.

Sadie, the 'baby' and her family

Although Sadie and 'baby' play the major role in the occurrence, I will highlight briefly some of the more pertinent observations with regard to Sadie, the doll and her son's reactions, drawing upon psychodynamic theory. Sadie's son presents as a very angry man. He used the nursing staff as a sounding board to vent his feelings of frustration, anxiety, and anger. Often as nurses we have no way of knowing exactly what is going on in people's minds, other than through their behaviour. He may have felt guilt at having little involvement with either of his parents or his sister in their times of need, or he may have felt real fear at seeing his mother like this, seemingly out of touch, in a fantasy state, and totally dependent. He focused on the doll, as this set his mother apart, and those who gave it to her were blamed for doing so. His intense rage may have developed from fear, as a number of relatives in my experience believe they too will develop the illness their parent has.

He may have been unconsciously expelling his own vulnerability and fear by projecting this into the ward sister, forcing her to withdraw the use of the doll. He used the same tactics on me, but instead of giving in, I stood my ground, however frightened I felt. McGhie (1979) describes such phenomena as the unconscious defence mechanism of 'projection', whereby Sadie's son projected his feelings into us. Erikson (1995, p. 223) suggests that projection is one of our deepest and most dangerous defence mechanisms, suggesting it is like 'experiencing an inner harm as an outer one: we endow significant people with the evil which actually is in us'. I was frightened by this man and maybe I was picking up his fear, or merely reacting to his aggression and hostility. What may have happened, from a psychodynamic perspective, was that the projected feelings were held by me, then reflected back, after they had been dealt with, thought about and processed in a manner made acceptable and plausible for him to tolerate, thus minimising his anxiety.

Menzies Lyth (1988) suggests nurses are expected unconsciously to receive and deal with projected feelings such as anxiety as part of their working day. This is to prevent patients and relatives from having to feel them, or at least to have them minimised. Sadie's son was an example of this expectation. Sister felt it easier to back off, but I felt it necessary to confront him, on Sadie's behalf and attempt to contain the situation. He needed to be emotionally held, or contained (like Winnicott's [1988] 'good enough' mother 'holding' the baby) in order to allow him the space to decide what was actually right for his mother, rather than focusing on how she looked. He needed to be helped to contribute to her well-being and care, something he may not have found possible previously. He was now given the power to do this. The reparative function undertaken by releasing this power, possibly served to relieve the guilt and anxiety displayed by the son. The gathering up of the fragments at the end of the occurrence is almost symbolic of the piecing together of Sadie's slowly disinte-grating mind, and the remnants of our nursing team.

'Baby', Sadie and nursing

Kitwood (1997) highlights common anxieties felt by those caring for people with dementia as fears of 'ageing, frailty, madness, and loss of self, with the additional threat that this might be me someday' (p.114). This is echoed by Skogstad (1997) who refers to occupational threats in nursing of contagion, not merely physically but also psychologically, leading to fears that nurses too, may become infected by unwanted feelings such as anxiety, helplessness, despair, fear, and fear of death. Dartington (1993, p. 31) supports this suggestion, claiming that emotional dependency is experienced as the most dangerous and contagious of diseases. Sometimes these fears are overwhelming and projected outside to free oneself of worry, as is the case when the contagion anxieties felt by those caring for people with dementia become so overwhelming they are dealt with by partially denying the human status of the sufferer.

With this in mind it is clear why some nursing staff felt strongly about Sadie being allowed the doll and some denied her this right. Bowlby and Murray Parkes (1970) suggest that in some families, attachment behaviour in a child is considered babyish and something to be grown out of as quickly as possible. It would follow that people of this belief could not condone an adult woman portraying such behaviour. However, interestingly, later on, all the nursing staff rallied round to protect Sadie from the potential removal of the doll by her son's threats because they had witnessed the distress caused and the behavioural consequences.

Conclusion

Recounting and analysing these events has highlighted the importance of purposeful reflective thought in nursing. Nurses, while actively caught up in the process of providing care, can find they have little time left to consider thinking about what they are doing and the impact it may have. In Sadie's case, applying psychodynamic theory to assist understanding of events has resulted in developing a substantial theory to support why the doll 'baby' was so important. Initially, nursing staff assumed it was merely regression which is fairly common in this field of care. However, this was not an adequate explanation for Sadie's behaviour.

It would appear that people with dementia can and do form new attachments and as part of this have the potential to draw others into their illusionary situation as in Sadie's case with nursing staff. The 'aliveness' of the doll in Sadie's eyes gave it a new meaning for those around her, once they were convinced of its importance. Sadie made this happen, as nursing staff we then advocated positively on her behalf. This may have been in the interest of self preservation, as indeed staff caring for Sadie found her far more amenable with 'baby' as opposed to without. However, I prefer to think it was from a fundamental respect of persons with dementia, gained by having had the privilege to practice in this field.

References

Bowlby, J. (1969). 'Affectional bonds: their nature and origin.' In *Progress in Mental Health: Proceedings of the Seventh International Congress on Mental Health*, ed. H. Freeman. London: J. and A. Churchill, pp. 319–27.

Bowlby, J. & Murray Parkes, C. (1970). 'Separation and loss within the family.' In *The Child in his Family. International Yearbook of Child Psychiatry and Allied Professions*, Vol. 1, eds. E.J. Anthony and C. Koupernik. New York: John Wiley, pp.197–215.

Bretherton, I. (1991). 'The roots and growing points of attachment theory.' In *Attachment Across the Life Cycle*, eds. C.M. Parkes, J. Stevenson-Hinde and P. Marris. London: Routledge, pp. 9–32.

Dartington, A. (1993). 'Where angels fear to tread: idealism, despondency, and inhibition in thought in hospital nursing.' *Winnicott Studies* 7, Spring: 21–41.

Erikson, E. H. (1995). *Childhood and Society.* London: Vintage.

Gomez, L. (1997). *An Introduction to Object Relations.* London: Free Association Press.

Gross, R.D. (1991). *Psychology: The Science of Mind and Behaviour.* London: Hodder and Stoughton.

Kitwood, T. (1997). *Dementia Reconsidered: The Person Comes First.* Buckingham: Open University Press.

Klein, M. (1963). *Our Adult World and Other Essays.* London: William Heinemann.

McGhie, A. (1979). *Psychology as Applied to Nursing.* 7th edn. Edinburgh: Churchill Livingstone.

Menzies Lyth, I. (1988). *Containing Anxiety in Institutions: Selected Essays*, Vol.1. London: Free Association Books.

Miesen, B. (1992). 'Attachment theory and dementia.' In *Care Giving in Dementia: Research and Applications*, eds. G. Jones and B. Miesen. London: Routledge, pp. 38–56.

Nichols, K.A. (1993). *Psychological Care in Physical Illness*, 2nd edn. London: Chapman and Hall.

Skogstad, W. (1997). 'Working in a world of bodies: defensive techniques on a medical ward – a psychoanalytical observation.' *Psychoanalytic Psychotherapy* 11(3): 221–41.

Winnicott, D.W. (1958). *Collected Papers: Through Paediatrics to Psycho-Analysis.* London: Tavistock Publications.

Winnicott, D.W. (1988). 'Breast-feeding as communication.' In *Babies and Their Mothers*. London: Free Association Books, pp. 23–49.

Commentary on 'Sadie's baby'
Mic Rafferty

This case study uses developmental ideas to present a sensitive interpretation of the experience of an old woman with dementia, which aids understanding and insight. It results from a retrospective, reflective activity about the care of this woman and seeks to validate the care given.

It is worth considering the background context of this chapter and the wider implications it has for this patient group. It is important to have insights into the dementia experience, given its incidence. The Medical Research Council (2005) estimate that there will be approximately one hundred and sixty-three thousand new cases of dementia occurring each year in England and Wales. The dementia experience is increasingly recognised as a 'long journey', with care and treatment able to make significant improvements, as a result of attitude change, skilled, well-resourced care and pharmacology breakthroughs, thereby pushing back the stereotype of dementia as 'living death'. We are now beginning to know more about the early experience of dementia, as those with the condition, for instance, the (now sadly deceased) musician, George Melley and the writer, Terry Pratchett, are prepared to make public their diagnosis and the nature of their experience. While such accounts provide insights that are both human and inspirational, for instance, Pratchett's belief that he has two more books in him, inevitably it is a journey about losses, fragmentation and anxiety. Therefore, the understanding about the experience of Sadie, contained in the chapter, should shed light on psychosocial issues relevant to all stages of the dementia journey.

The care story revolves around the interpretation of Sadie's experience that arose out of the need to find a way to deal with her aggressive reactions to intimate care. The doll, a longstanding strategy used by the family to get Sadie's cooperation, was found to be the answer. Central to the story are the strong feelings of others about what is right and proper behaviour, with those having negative reactions to the doll seeing it as inappropriate, infantile and demeaning of Sadie's status. This demonstrates the situation of vulnerability that elderly people with advanced dementia are in, as they are open to the projections of others as to what is needed, what is to be allowed and what discounted. Such patients are unlikely to be able to directly challenge these interpretations.

The study provides insights about this institutional care setting, and the degree to which it has the characteristics of an open or closed system. Closed institutional systems tend to be cut off from the wider community, with regimented routines and a lack of emphasis on patient individuality, thereby enhancing the patient's experience of being 'sans everything' (George Orwell, 1918, cited by Stansky and Abrahams, 1994). No privacy, no choice, no meaningful activity or recreation is likely to enhance the disintegration of the individual. Open systems, on the other hand, are characterised by their openness to the input and influence of other systems, as shown by the fact that Sadie's family were actively involved in her care. In addition, the ward staff were able to entertain a lively conversation about the wisdom of incorporating the doll, as part of the plan of care, showing that they were able to risk ambiguity, in that more than one explanation could be tolerated. Importantly, this ward system also had the capacity to give Sadie the status of an individual, by remembering her individual need for the doll, thereby gaining her cooperation by reducing her fear of being taken over, particularly when undressed and naked.

Central to the study is the use of psychodynamic ideas, particularly about transitional phenomena, to examine the meaning of a doll for Sadie. It captures a moment in Sadie's life when she is dealing with multiple losses: loss of her deceased husband and of intimate contact, loss of her home, of her daughter's care and the presence of the family. In addition, Sadie is dealing with the losses which result from dementia, which affect all aspects of life from memory to relationship quality.

Miesen (1992) characterises the dementia experience as provoking in the patient something similar to the stranger-situation for the young infant, who responds anxiously, and searchingly for their attachment figure, to provide the secure base to deal with a feeling of insecurity. Importantly for the person with end stage dementia, the stranger-situation and resulting anxiety never ends. As identified in this case study, any explanation of the meaning of Sadie's behaviour has at its heart her indomitable spirit and drive to create a secure base to deal with her predicament. Such drive and spirit capture well the psychoanalytic truth that, given a facilitating environment, we seek development, typified by the idea of again being 'a going concern' (Winnicott, 1964, p. 25).

It is worth considering that all the explanations of Sadie's behaviour with the doll are rooted in transitional phenomena, as a way of managing anxiety. As Grace Sansom ably demonstrates, this understanding makes it more possible to understand how Sadie used a transitional object (the doll) to confidently manage anxiety-inducing transitions, such as being undressed and washed (Winnicott, 1958).

Winnicott (1958), following observations of young children and their mothers, began to look at the psychic significance to infants of their special things (for instance a special blanket, toy, or a bedtime routine), and the ways they were used for comfort and soothing. He argued that such things were transitional phenomena, in that they enabled the infant to cope with anxiety-provoking transitions, such as moving from waking to sleeping, going from place to place (home to school), or being able to separate from their primary attachment figure. Winnicott argued that all transitional phenomena are invested with tacit affectional links, such as a special blanket, which becomes a patchwork quilt of sensations, memories and smells, related to the child's parents, themselves and their environment. At a primitive, unconscious level, Winnicott argued that transitional phenomena first begin to appear with the infant's beginning comprehension that they are separate from their mother and most importantly do not control her. The anxiety that this provokes leads the infant towards having a transitional object, something special and comforting, 'whose' absence and presence they can control. Such a 'not me' and 'not mother' object, in the safe routines of care becomes invested with feelings of security, comfort and control.

Winnicott suggests that transitional phenomena are found in all ages of life, from lucky charms, to the 'leaving home' routines enacted before a journey. It is also worth noting that transitional phenomena are important sources of a sense of self and the ability to rely on self. For instance transitional objects have a root in parental encouragement for a child to develop its own soothers, in order to develop the capacity to be self-reliant (for example, 'Go and play…'). In adult life, such transitional phenomena can include cultural and religious activities, such as praying, enjoying music and art (Winnicott, 1958, p. 233).

Grace captures well in her work, the special qualities of transitional phenomena described by Winnicott, and seeks to determine which of them was applicable to Sadie's doll. Her thinking about the unconscious use of the doll, to enact Sadie's assumptive world of purpose, that is to care for children, also implied that this acted as an emblem of her past, for the staff. This came to be seen as an expression of Sadie's individuality, ultimately gaining her respect. Even in her aggression, Sadie typifies Winnicott's idea that resistant and rebellious actions are protests and pleas for a facilitating environment, to make anxiety-inducing transitions possible. The staff, through being constantly confronted by her 'rock bottom' attitude of defiance when the doll was absent, learnt (self protectively) never to change or lose it again, in the service of Sadie's individuality.

Grace also identifies that the aliveness that came to Sadie in her interactions with the doll, awakened in her a protective caretaker response. This is attachment behaviour. She was prepared to challenge the son's angry assertion that the doll was a demeaning infantilisation of his mother. Grace was able to survive the son's hateful reaction to the doll and negotiate with him a more loving understanding of the purpose of the doll for his mother's welfare. Grace sadly points to the fact that the transitional object (the doll) could never offer a bridge to development, as Sadie was stuck in the fragmented and declining world of dementia. Such a view could be more hopefully recast, to suggest that the developmental imperative still operated in Sadie, even if this was limited. Through having control of her doll, Sadie was able to create an environment in which she could reveal her ability to be content and alive, rather than fraught and anxious.

References

Miesen, B. (1992). 'Attachment theory and dementia.' In *Care Giving in Dementia: Research and Applications*, eds. G. Jones and B. Miesen. London: Routledge, pp. 38–56.

Stansky, P. and Abrahams, W. (1994). *The Unknown Orwell and Orwell*. San Francisco: Stanford University Press.

The Medical Research Council (2005). Cognitive Function and Ageing Study. http://www.cfas.ac.uk/pages/incident/index.html (Accessed 4 August 2008)

Winnicott, D. (1958). 'Transitional objects and transitional phenomena.' In *Collected Papers: Through Paediatrics to Psychoanalysis*. London: Tavistock Publications, pp.229–42.

Winnicott, D. (1964). *The Child, the Family and the Outside World*. Harmondsworth: Penguin Books.

Chapter 9
Pre-operative anxiety: understanding why?
Wendy Kennedy

Introduction

A psychodynamic perspective of nursing offers important insights into my role as an anaesthetic and recovery nurse. My work involves high intensity, short duration relationships with people who are anxious and about whom I know nothing, except for their name, date of birth, hospital number, and the details of the proposed operation. It is therefore important to understand the nature of the anxiety in patients who enter the anaesthetic room, in order to improve practice and deliver quality patient care. Three clinical stories will demonstrate how everyday situations that nurses experience may subconsciously affect their practice. Attachment theory, social defence mechanisms and Winnicott's theory of transitional objects may help explain nurses' responses to patients.

When faced with the prospect of having to undergo surgery many patients find the thought of the experience terrifying (see Chapter 3). Although it may be argued that anxiety is a form of protection that triggers alarm (Selye, 1956), well-documented evidence supports the notion that increased pre-operative anxiety may have a detrimental effect on recovery following surgery (Allcock, 1986, Mitchell, 1994, Coleman and White, 2001). One role of the anaesthetic nurse is to understand and manage patient anxiety in order to have a positive outcome. Pre-operative visiting by anaesthetic nurses from the operating department has been demonstrated to help patients overcome their fears of surgery (Reid, 1998, Coleman and White, 2001) enabling theatre staff to meet their patients, provide information and give reassurance, all methods for decreasing anxiety (Hayward, 1975, Boore, 1978).

However, despite this research evidence, only a small percentage of patients receive a pre-operative visit. The reasons for this apparent non-utilisation of research include staff shortages and lack of time. Examining this from a psychodynamic perspective and from the nurses' position, could it be fear of intolerable anxiety that leads to a social system's defence which becomes the unconscious reason for the failure of pre-operative visiting? For example, by not getting involved, nurses are avoiding emotional involvement, albeit at a sub-conscious level.

The first clinical story involves a student nurse and examines whether attachment theory can be used to explain aspects of an adult patient's reactions in times of heightened anxiety, and whether nurses can be viewed as transitional objects (Winnicott, 1951). Such ideas may help to explain patients' responses to illness, and inform practice.

First story: attachment

Attachment

During an elective surgical list, a patient arrived in the anaesthetic room visibly shaking, head bowed, and very tense. My initial reaction was of surprise; even though I am used to seeing visible signs of anxiety, this patient seemed petrified. The patient was accompanied by a student nurse, much younger than herself, who asked if it would be alright to stay with the patient until she was anaesthetised. The student nurse was clearly acting on behalf of the patient, as the lady gestured to her to ask. Although I was taken aback by such an unusual request when an adult was involved (although normal for children), I confirmed that it was fine. To help understand the situation, it is important to examine how my feelings contributed to the way I responded to this patient, as the nurse–patient relationship is a two-way process, with the actions and responses of one ultimately affecting the other.

Views on what motivates human action have emanated from a belief that our actions are determined by conscious experience. However Freud (2001, original paper 1923) suggests that unconscious mechanisms have a great influence on conscious life, illustrated by human responses to grief, where denial is an unconscious response to loss (see Chapters 1 and 3). The loss may be physical (loss of a spouse) or triggered by deep anxiety. Freud

Pre-operative anxiety: understanding why?

(2001) maintained that part of our mind contained thoughts and feelings, far beyond the conscious level (the unconscious) and suggested that the unconscious contained thoughts that at one time had been available at a conscious level, but were later repressed, into the unconscious. McGhie (1979) refers to such stimuli that are received deep into our unconscious, as subliminal cues. Such feelings being brought to a conscious level have implications for nurses.

Initially, on meeting the patient, my interest in 'knowing' the patient was founded on a professional wish for a relationship in which the patient can (in a very short space of time) trust me. Trust at this level is multi-faceted and open-ended, but needs to be developed so the patient can feel safe. For example, it may involve the need to talk, or sometimes just to be there and reassure the patient. For the patient, this is a situation of vulnerability, for coming to the operating theatre entails leaving a known ward environment and nurses they know and entering the care of a different team of people whom they probably have not met. For many people, having an operation not only conjures up fears of death (Robertson, 1957) but also fears of being anaesthetised, of pain and discomfort, and of the operation itself, as well as of being unconscious (Mitchell, 2000). The surgical procedure may be to cure an illness, or confirm a diagnosis that will change their life forever. Therefore, for the patient, the experience is at the very least uncomfortable psychologically (even the most laid-back individual has some feelings of trepidation) as it can herald a transition that has psychosocial implications of huge proportions. Therefore, for the patient entering the anaesthetic room, the experience may signify all manner of emotions, including loss, grief or hope.

At first I felt this person was overreacting, and I could have acted on such feelings, in a belief that I knew something about the patient, by making such a judgement. Munhall (1993) claims that 'knowing' in such a way may lead to 'closure' as the nurse gains false confidence in her interpretation of experience. However, drawing on the philosophical definition of knowledge as justified, true belief, my feelings about the patient could not be taken as knowledge. I as an individual had no means of differentiating between accurate and inaccurate feelings, without being able to check them out. Therefore, to remain 'unknowing' was a more appropriate position. Heath (1998) describes 'unknowing' as an:

> … awareness that the nurse does not and cannot know or understand the client when they first meet, and by recognising this unknowing the nurse remains alert to the clients' perspective of the situation. (Heath, 1998, p.1057)

Watching the way the patient responded to the student nurse, and listening to their conversation, I was able to think through the whole situation, and keep an open mind as to the patient's needs. By taking this position, I was aware of my feelings, but used them to remain alert to their significance in understanding the patient's perspective of the situation.

I experienced mixed feelings; although I tried to relieve the patient's anxiety by reassurance, I felt almost redundant, as the existing relationship between the patient and the nurse was very apparent. Their conversation indicated that the patient had talked to the student at length about her life, discussing holidays and family matters. There appeared to be no room for me in their relationship; however, I also felt pleased that the patient had such a good rapport with the student, at a time when she was most vulnerable. I was surprised at my mixed feelings and the feeling of being 'left out' I attributed to an unconscious expression of a childish reaction. I realised that there was no room for such feelings, and therefore the 'adult self' accepted the situation, and no issue was made. I quickly realised that it was important to 'let things be', as the relationship with the student nurse was in fact potentially helpful for the patient.

I had alternative courses of action open to me. I could have rejected the student nurse's request to stay, unable to cope with the jealousy of another person taking my place. It is possible that another nurse may have taken exception to the student nurse making such a request; after all nursing has a tradition of being rigidly hierarchical. Maintaining such a position would not have helped the patient, and is an illustration of how personal feelings can have a detrimental effect on patient care.

I was unable to establish my usual relationship with the patient, although this did highlight for me the importance of the role in developing a helping relationship with very anxious patients. I focused attention on the technical aspect of the role, such as attaching vital sign monitors. Although technical and routine, its effect on the patient cannot be underestimated, as many patients find this experience alarming, with others finding comfort in knowing they are going to be monitored throughout the procedure. Jarvis (1992, p. 178) warns about actions that require minimal thought becoming 'mindless alienation' from the situation, or being on 'auto-pilot'. This has the potential to become destructive, if not recognised. The patient, anxious at being in a new environment, requires the nurse to focus on them. It is possible that nurses use the repetitive nature of some tasks as a way of not engaging with the patient, a form of distraction to prevent them getting too involved. To reassure the patient that I was receptive to her anxiety, I explained the reason for the monitoring, what vital sign each machine monitored, and assured her that she was in safe hands. She seemed reluctant to accept my reassurances (looking away towards the student who was now holding her hand) but reinforcement by the student was accepted. Such simple explanations can have a positive effect on reducing anxiety (Teasdale, 1995, Mitchell, 2000).

At this juncture, I could have withdrawn from any further attempts to communicate with my patient and become preoccupied with technical routine tasks. However, I felt that I still needed to gain her trust, as the student would soon have to leave the patient in my care and return to the ward. I realised I would have to change tack and attempt to work together with the student to find ways to engage with the patient. I now needed to 'nurse the couple' (Weddell, 1968) to enable the patient to undergo a smooth transition into my care, allowing the student to feel that her task had been accomplished before returning to the ward. Any other action may have resulted in alienation of the student who may have felt helpless leaving her patient. I was sub-consciously preparing the student for leaving the patient in my care.

In childhood, parents are normally the main figures of attachment, and Bowlby (1971) referred to them as providing a 'secure base' from which to explore the world. Bowlby maintained that attachment behaviour can be reawakened in adult life, when the attachment figure may be any person who is believed to be able to offer protection from a perceived threat (Bowlby, 1971). Bowlby (1971) argued that humans and other animals have developed systems which enable adaptation to and offer protection from the environment. One form of attachment behaviour is the response to a perceived threat which draws a response from an attachment figure willing to come to one's aid. This is an example of someone undertaking a 'caretaker' role when we perceive that we are not going to be in control and are therefore vulnerable, thus unconsciously confirming that the biological function of attachment behaviour is protection from predators.

The physical presence of a nurse or relative during a stressful event has been proven to be of great benefit to the patient (Robertson 1957, Leinonen *et al.* 1996). Similarly, if an anxious patient regards the nurse as a powerful figure, who is able and willing to give protection from the fears of threat to integrity that imminent surgery might provoke, attachment theory suggests that the presence of the nurse will induce the patient to feel calmer and more secure. Furthermore, it may be that under certain circumstances, nurses may be able to reassure their patients by their very presence. This can be compared to the reassuring presence of a parent for a young child; when the parent goes out of a room the child becomes fretful. Bowlby (1975) referred to such a reaction as separation anxiety. Vogelsang (1990) established that continued contact with one nurse helped to achieve a similar consequence. That is, having the same nurse from pre-assessment clinic through to discharge on the day of surgery, improved satisfaction with care and led to an earlier discharge.

How then can attachment theory be used to explain the relationship between the student nurse and this patient, given the unusual intensity of the relationship? In order to answer the question, much of my argument is based on my interpretation of what had happened on the ward, as I was not there and can only surmise. The relationship between my patient and the student may have been construed as intense. In my experience it was certainly an extreme example of anxiety in one person and their dependence on another, who was not related. We can presume that the patient would be aware of the nurse as a separate entity (not related) who was being paid to do a job in a hospital. As already discussed, illness itself can cause regression and may be understood as a method of coping with the reality of present difficulties (hospitalisation, impending diagnostic surgery, and fear) by returning to a previous less mature way of adjusting to an intolerable, anxiety-inducing situation (McGhie, 1979, p. 180). Regression provokes dependency and summons a need for an attachment figure. In a sense the patient created for herself a needed other, with the student prepared to be that person. This idea has its limits, as nurses cannot be everything their patients want them to be, as the nurse has self-limits as to what is acceptable. A further example from my practice illustrates this concept.

Second story: boundaries

Boundaries

Another aspect of my role involves hand-holding for patients undergoing cataract surgery; such physical contact provides an avenue for non-verbal communication and may be a great source of comfort and a relief from anxiety. Using attachment theory, we are aware of the security and comfort a child gains from handholding when unsure or frightened. Most of the time, patients take my hand for the duration of the case, though occasionally male patients make comments of a flirtatious nature, which I laugh off and make light of. On one occasion, the patient had been given a local anaesthetic, and the surgeon had told him that I would hold his hand. At this point, the patient grabbed my hand and made obvious sexual insinuations in his actions and verbally. I withdrew my hand and told him that he must not do that, as I would not be able to tell if he required help during the procedure.

I maintained reality by reminding the patient of my role, and the reason for the contact, as opposed to getting confused by the patient's sexual fantasies/ideas. If I had not done that, I would have been no use to the patient at that time. My reaction was one of shock that he had felt that he could take advantage of my professional requirement to have physical contact with him, resulting in my not wanting to hold his hand at all. As a nurse, although not prepared to be exploited, I could not bring myself to sit there and not hold his hand. When the procedure started, I held his hand without issue, but as soon as possible I asked a male nursing auxiliary to take my place. This patient appeared to need someone to take on an intimate and sexual role, as a response to his anxiety, raising awareness that some of the more 'intimate' things that nurses have to do for people may provoke excitement or a misreading of the situation in a susceptible person. Such conversion of fear into excitement is common and can be described as a manic defence, but it may also be provoked or intensified by the stimulation of physical contact and its associations.

Transitional phenomena

Transitional phenomena

Returning to the student nurse and my patient, attachment theory can explain her need for someone being there, as attachment behaviour is a normal human response that occurs through life, in response to threat. It may be useful to examine whether deeper unconscious thoughts and experiences are also motivators for human responses. Winnicott's (1951) theory of transitional objects and transitional phenomena may explain such reactions to illness. Winnicott (1951) describes the time in the middle of the child's developing capacity to differentiate between what is 'me' (for example, the thumb) and what is 'not me' (for example, the teddy bear); this links to earlier experiences of breast feeding. A baby's first experience is usually of the mother's breast, though the baby has no way of differentiating this from itself, to a baby it is simply an extension of the self. Winnicott (1988) maintains that the act of feeding is vital for psychosocial development, as it is the way in which the mother brings an awareness of the outside world to her child. Winnicott (1988) terms this 'object presenting'. Done well, the baby is ready to receive and explore, with the mother allowing increasing independence, stemming from such experiences as letting the baby find the nipple rather than having it thrust at it. This idea extends to reaching for a toy, sucking the thumb, burble and smile responses. The baby is creating his world, of oneness and separateness and making connections to others. As babies develop, they begin to realise that they are separate from the outside world, it is 'not me'. The thumb as 'me' begins to be distinguished from other objects which are 'not me'.

Winnicott (1951) sees this as an intermediate state between the inability and a growing ability to recognise and accept reality. Thus the transitional object creates an illusion of control, in a world where the baby has little control. As a means of dealing with such an intermediate state of experience, a baby may become attached to an object, for example teddy bear or blanket, which, though recognised as 'not me', is imbued with some 'part-object' association, such as the breast. However, the baby knows the teddy or blanket is not the breast or the mother, thereby distinguishing between fantasy and fact, but nevertheless vital importance is still attached to these things, especially in times of need, when tired, anxious, or upset. Such patterns may endure into childhood, becoming less needed with a gradual widening of interests, so the need for the object diminishes, even under the threat of anxiety.

Winnicott (1951) argues that even in adult life, a need for a specific object or type of behaviour may reappear. As adults, in health, we allow ourselves to slip in and out of reality, which may be an extension of the 'me-not-me' concept, and at intervals we seem to operate in a transitional space in between the two. When we go to see a play or a film, we sit and enjoy the story line, and enter fully into it, as if it were real. We become immersed and consequently lose a sense of reality and for that period of time, reality is not a concern, and in a sense, we are enjoying transitional space phenomena, much as might be experienced by babies. How then can this be applied to a nursing situation?

Transference and transitional phenomena

Transference

For the woman in the anaesthetic room the student nurse became what she needed. It may have been that the patient unconsciously regressed to behaviour from childhood, to cope with her distress and anxiety, but there may also be a valid link with Winnicott's (1951) ideas. The notion of transference may help to explain this. O'Kelly (1998) describes transference as: '... an unconscious process in which a person displaces, feelings, thoughts, and behaviours originally experienced in relation to significant figures in the past to a current relationship' (O'Kelly, 1998, p. 392).

This patient, therefore, may have used the student nurse as a maternal transference object, projecting on to her unconscious feelings associated with her mother. In a similar way, the man undergoing cataract surgery may have made me into a transference figure of a wife or a lover, in response to anxiety, and fear of the operation. Winnicott (1951) makes no claim that a person can have projected upon them unconscious feelings, similar to those a child has for a transitional object, but are we able to consciously separate reality and unreality in times of intense anxiety? If we do not question reality when enjoying a film and if the transitional object is indeed a part-object symbolising the breast, then is it not also feasible that a person, may, in the same way become a symbol for a mother figure, in association with a transference. Such processes take place deep in our unconscious minds and may not be available as 'thoughts'. If Winnicott (1951) is correct in suggesting that wider interests may mean that the transitional object is no longer required, maybe it is relationships with other people that start to fill the gap. Although not an object such as a blanket or a teddy bear, a person and what they signify may become similarly as important as a transitional object.

Dependence

Dependence

In the nursing situation, dependence may result in emotional involvement with potentially harmful consequences for the patient. For example, depending on the nurse may delay the patient taking responsibility for their own recovery (Petri and Weinman, 1997). The nurse may avoid such situations, putting up defensive barriers, which could interfere with a positive experience for the patient. Regarding the first story, an initial impression was that the student's involvement suggested an element of dependence by the patient. Such a relationship may increase patient anxiety and result in the patient not being adequately psychologically prepared for theatre. If this dependence was for a short period of time, and ended and resolved in the post-operative phase, into a more adult and equal involvement, then such a relationship could only serve a positive outcome. Through such a relationship, the patient would have had less anxiety and felt more comfortable with the thought of her operation, and coming to theatre.

Such a junior nurse may experience feelings of being 'out of her depth' in trying to deal with dependence. She may not have thought to ask for professional help and support from more experienced staff. Without support networks, there is a risk of loss of professional confidence and withdrawal from the patient.

Therefore, it is not the dependency that causes harm but the inability of nurses to deal with it, once recognised. For the nurse, responding to patient attachment behaviour may mean costs in both time and personal investment, as it requires a relationship, affection and therefore involvement.

One can only wonder whether the other ward nurses may have been wary of forming what appeared to be a close, dependent relationship with the patient. Such feelings may arise from confusing attachment with dependence behaviour. If the view is held that attachment has time and emotional costs, resulting from possible affection and involvement, coupled with the conviction that this may lead to dependence, it might explain many nurses' reluctance to give emotional and psychological space to their patients. However, if by considering attachment theory and then taking the position that it is an innate human response that is heightened by hospitalisation and states of anxiety, with regression being inevitable, the nurse may accept that being there physically and emotionally for the patient, is in fact helpful, and can aid recovery.

The student nurse was prepared to establish such a relationship, and enabled a smooth transition from ward to theatre for the patient. It is possible that a qualified nurse would have been less receptive to this patient's needs for an attachment figure. Both clinical stories demonstrate the intense emotional nature of theatre nursing and how avoidance of involvement by nurses gives a possible reason why pre-operative visiting has not been developed by theatre nurses. The avoidance of involvement may be a defence mechanism used to prevent anxiety. Such a defence is a way of avoiding having to think about the anxieties that each individual experiences pre-operatively. By not visiting, the nurse does not have to become contaminated by a patient's suffering, bad news, or the threat of death which some operative procedures herald. Similarly, might the ward staff have allowed the student nurse to take on such a role, as it relieved them of the burden of having to get involved with the patient's anxieties?

Referring to patients by their surgical procedure may illustrate the wish not to get too involved. To the nurse a label may be easier to acknowledge and understand, than the complexities of what the procedure really means to the patient. The role of the anaesthetic nurse allows time and there is an expectation that patient anxieties should be recognised (the time element may be more problematical in other clinical settings within the demands of the current NHS). However, without the social systems in place to support nurses' emotional needs, it is little wonder that nurses adopt mechanisms of protection for themselves. Allowing the student to go to theatre was perhaps a means of concrete protection for the qualified nurses. Skogstad (1997) conducted an observational study on a medical ward of a busy hospital. He concluded that nursing generates anxiety in nurses, due to the nature of the work which very often reminds us of our own mortality, or provokes feelings of guilt when faced with suffering that we cannot do more to relieve. An illustration follows.

The third story: life and death

Life and death

Recently, a patient arrived in the anaesthetic room in a life-threatening, critical condition, with the success of the operation meaning the difference between life and death. She was particularly well and chatty, in spite of her condition, and fully aware of what was going on around her. Due to the nature of her illness, it was necessary to anaesthetise her on the operating table, which meant she had to be positioned, exposed, cleansed and draped before anaesthesia was administered. To undergo such procedures must be one of the most terrifying experiences; to realise that surgeons are ready, the minute you become unconscious. I held her hand and stroked her face, as I felt this was the only comfort I could give her. The look in her eyes portrayed helplessness and fear, until her eyes closed. In such an operation everyone is kept busy, the atmosphere is one of almost manic work. In the middle of this life saving procedure, the surgeon stood back and said: 'I cannot do any more, I can't stop the bleeding'. I wanted to say: 'But you have to, you can't just walk away and let her die,' but that is what had to happen. I felt useless, and inadequate, I felt that I had let her down, and it did cause me anxiety, until I had thought about my feelings, and talked to my colleagues.

This is just one example of how nursing work causes anxiety, and it is little wonder that nurses use defence mechanisms against it. However, defence mechanisms could be adaptive, provided one recognised how to use them in such a way. As mentioned earlier, reflecting on such feelings and experience, and thus being prepared, can positively affect the nurse–patient relationship. Such reflection and discussion may be addressed by clinical supervision either formally (ideally) or informally. Menzies Lyth (1988) maintains that collective defence mechanisms may be employed by people who work together (for example, labelling the patient, as mentioned above). She suggests that the over-use of such primitive defence mechanisms results in the loss of reality. It is important for nurses to keep hold of some feeling for the patient as an individual, and maintain a caring relationship rather than immersing themselves in work (keeping busy) to reduce anxiety. It would be very easy for an anaesthetic nurse to put monitoring on a patient without using it as an opportunity to address patient anxiety. Such actions become task oriented, without meaning, which pays lip service to total patient care.

Conclusion

This chapter has attempted to understand why pre-operative visiting is neglected by some nurses in some Trusts, and has concluded that it may be due to the defence mechanisms that nurses may employ (sub-consciously) to avoid the anxiety provoked by attachment and the perceived dependence that may result. Furthermore, by examining the psychodynamic perspectives linked to attachment, anxiety, and unconscious motivation, some empowering ideas have been suggested that could be useful in helping nurses understand the nurse–patient relationship. Indeed, scientific subjectivity based on emotional and subjective evidence could be used as a valuable source of new nursing knowledge, and thus inform practice (Skogstad, 1997). Certainly the clinical stories relating to the anaesthetic room illustrate this point. The anaesthetic room is based on science (monitors and anaesthetic equipment), but using it well ensures that each patient's emotional needs are met.

The ideas raised are merely suggestions that could answer the question of why pre-operative visiting is not more widespread, despite research proving its worth. Is it part of a defence mechanism at work in nursing? Could it be addressed by improved support systems in place for nurses? It is up to the reader to decide if the explanations suggested are plausible. If I had not read about and examined the concept of psychodynamic perspectives in nursing, I would not have considered what motivates my actions, and the importance of the concepts mentioned. I consider myself better informed for exploring how attachment and Winnicott's (1951) theory of transitional objects may unconsciously motivate my patients, and how I react to them.

I believe that the explanations given are plausible, but care should be taken not to use such ideas prescriptively. It is up to the individual to decide if they are able or prepared to examine their deepest feelings, which can consequently inform practice. Increasing our own self-awareness by addressing the issues is a starting point. With the pre-operative patient, nurses should give the patient opportunities to disclose their fears, rather than quietening them with reassurance. The nurse thus communicates acceptance of them, as genuine fears, as distinct from suggesting that they are unrealistic. Enabling patients to verbalise their genuine fears may promote a more active and less helpless attitude. Being there for the patient in such a way makes it necessary to be prepared to put aside one's own anxieties, and have an understanding of what motivates action, and to work with patients by trying to understand them.

Patients in hospital experience many emotions linked with hospitalisation, threat of illness and its subsequent meanings, and are not in control of what happens to them. They meet many people, endure transfer of care from one department to another, and from one health professional to another. By examining three patient–nurse encounters it has been possible to demonstrate the importance of considering nursing from a psychodynamic perspective, with the implication that nurses be invited to develop awareness of their feelings, in order to understand their motivation for caring for others.

References

Allcock, P. (1986). 'Pre-operative information and visits promote the recovery of patients.' *NATN News* 23: 17—18.

Boore, J.R.P. (1978). *Prescription for Recovery*. London: Royal College of Nursing.

Pre-operative anxiety: understanding why?

Bowlby, J. (1971). *Attachment*, Vol. 1 of *Attachment and Loss*. Harmondsworth: Penguin.

Bowlby, J. (1975). *Separation: Anxiety and Anger*, Vol. 2 of *Attachment and Loss*. Harmondsworth: Penguin.

Coleman, M. and White, J. (2001). 'Preoperative visiting in Wales: a study of its prevalence and nature.' *Nursing Times Research* 6(11): 611–25.

Freud, S. (2001). 'The ego and the id' [1923]. In *The Standard Edition of the Complete Works of Sigmund Freud*, Vol. X1X. London: Vintage, pp. 3–66.

Hayward, J. (1975). *Information: a Prescription against Pain*. London: Royal College of Nursing.

Heath, H. (1998). 'Reflection and patterns of knowing in nursing.' *Journal of Advanced Nursing* 27(5): 1054–9.

Jarvis, P. (1992). 'Reflective practice and nursing.' *Nurse Education Today* 12: 174–81.

Leinonen, T., Leino-Kilpi, H. and Jouko, K. (1996). 'The quality of intra-operative nursing care: the patient's perspective.' *Journal of Advanced Nursing* 24(4): 843–52.

McGhie, A. (1979). *Psychology as Applied to Nursing*, 7th edn. Edinburgh: Churchill Livingstone.

Menzies Lyth, I. (1988). 'The functioning of social systems as a defence against anxiety.' In *Containing Anxiety in Institutions: Selected Essays*. London: Free Association Books.

Mitchell, M. (1994). 'Pre-operative and postoperative psychological nursing care.' *Surgical Nurse* 7(3): 22—5.

Mitchell, M. (2000). 'Nursing intervention for pre-operative anxiety.' *Nursing Standard* 14(37): 40–3.

Munhall, P.L. (1993). ' "Unknowing": toward another pattern of knowing in nursing.' *Nursing Outlook* 41: 125–8.

O'Kelly, G. (1998). 'Countertransference in the nurse-patient relationship: a review of the literature.' *Journal of Advanced Nursing* 28 (2): 391–7.

Petrie, K.J. and Weinman, J.A. (1997). *Perceptions of Health and Illness*. London: Harwood.

Reid, J.H. (1998). 'Pre-operative information giving: An essential element of peri-operative practice.' *British Journal of Theatre Nursing* 8(6): 27—9.

Robertson, J. (1957). 'A mother's observations on the tonsillectomy of her four-year-old daughter.' *Nursing Times* (15 November): 1295–307.

Selye, H. (1956). *The Stress of Life*. New York: McGraw Hill.

Skogstad, W. (1997). 'Working in a world of bodies, defensive techniques on a medical ward – a psychoanalytical observation.' *Psychoanalytic Psychotherapy* 11(3): 221–41.

Teasdale, K. (1995). 'Theoretical and practical considerations on the use of reassurance in the nursing management of anxious patients.' *Journal of Advanced Nursing* 22(1): 79–86.

Vogelsang, J. (1990). 'Continued contact with a familiar nurse affects women's perceptions of the ambulatory surgical experience: a qualitative-quantitative design.' *Journal of Post Anaesthetic Nursing* 5(5): 315–20.

Weddell, D. (1968). 'Family centred nursing.' In *Psychosocial Nursing: Studies from the Cassel Hospital*, ed. E. Barnes. London: Tavistock Publications, pp. 137–42.

Winnicott, D.W. (1951). 'Transitional objects and transitional phenomena' [1951]. In *Collected Papers: Through Paediatrics to Psycho-Analysis*. London: Tavistock Publications, pp. 229–42.

Winnicott, D.W. (1988). *Babies and Their Mothers*. London: Free Association Books.

Commentary on 'Pre-operative anxiety: understanding why?'

Mic Rafferty

The chapter is written from the perspective of an anaesthetic and recovery nurse concerned with understanding operation anxiety, and its relationship to unconscious responses. As the nurse–patient relationship is a significant mediator of pre-operative anxiety, which has post-operative outcome implications, understanding this is important.

A dimension of the chapter is about work-induced anxiety in nurses and the institutional social systems used to defend against such anxiety. The work of Menzies (1970) is used to argue that from a psychological viewpoint, organisational culture, structure and mode of functioning can be seen to be determined by the worker's psychological needs. Work culture, structure and ways of functioning create institutional defences, which collectively help individuals to deal with the threat of persecutory or depressive anxieties, resulting from caring for patients.

Klein's ideas about how the infant deals with depressive and persecutory anxieties by splitting and projective processes are central to understanding social system defences and the forms that they take. The ideas of Klein (1946) used by Jacques (1955) and Menzies (1970) to develop explanations of social system defences are complicated. Klein was concerned with understanding the early strategies operated by infants to deal with and explain states of contentment or intolerable distress. Following study of the early development of infants, she suggested that the central defence available to the infant was to

Commentary on 'Pre-operative anxiety'

split experiences into either good or bad, thereby almost creating alternative existences like heaven and hell. Klein employs the analogy of the mother's breasts, to illustrate the infantile way internal and external comfort and discomfort are seen to arise from a good or bad breast. When confronting discomfort resulting from the absence of relief, the infant may regard this as wilful and therefore persecutory, with discomfort understood to be imposed from outside and the fault of the bad breast. The good breast, given the sustenance and comfort it provides, becomes loved and idealised. Depressive anxieties arise from the frightening realisation, on the infant's part, that the good and bad breasts are aspects of the same person, that is mother can bring both comfort and frustration. Such persecutory and depressive anxieties provoke splitting (for instance idealisation or denigration), and projection. That is dealing with anxiety provoking thoughts, feelings, and wishes by unconsciously putting them into the other (see Chapters 1 and 4).

Such prototype, unconscious mental processes persist into adulthood, although developmental experience will determine how reliant any individual is upon finding the source of any discomfort as someone else's fault (persecutory) or their own fault (depressive). While this is a very simplistic explanation of Klein's ideas, it does hopefully do enough to show how such mental defences develop and in their most primitive form, how dangerous they can be, when used by individuals or groups. So, work-related anxiety leads to the development of socially structured defence mechanisms, which impact upon the structure, culture and functioning of the organisation to help avoid feelings of anxiety, guilt and uncertainty (Menzies, 1970, p. 10).

Menzies determined that nurses have to struggle to manage the anxieties inherent in the work, which result from vulnerability and accountability. In the 1960s, Menzies (1970, p.123) noticed that the social system defences among nurses in hospitals seemed designed to minimise anxieties related to individual and group vulnerability and responsibility. While much has changed in the nature of nursing since the 1970s, it is still possible to suggest, as Wendy Kennedy does, that the lack of uptake of pre-surgery visiting by theatre nurses could result from a social systems defence to avoid relationships centred on dependency or attachment. To support such an assertion, Wendy includes a clinical story about a woman who died on the table from haemorrhaging, and the personal distress that arose from a feeling of surgical failure, exacerbated by an experience of trusting intimacy with this patient, during preparation for anaesthesia. She implicitly concludes that getting close to patients can have an emotional cost; hence, the social system defences to guard against and avoid feelings of anxiety, guilt and uncertainty. Such conclusions are valid, as in clinical supervision, it is usual to work with nurses trying to deal with upset, arising out of meeting a patient's attachment need, during a fearful transition, which leads unexpectedly to death and leaves the nurse feeling a betrayer of the patient's trust.

A clinical illustration is about a petrified patient able to deal with her pre-surgical anxiety by latching on to a student nurse who is prepared to be the caretaker, by helping to keep 'hope alive' and offer containment, by a willingness to be present. Wendy asks if the inevitable naivety and willingness of the student nurse has been used by other nurses, who would find such a task of reassurance daunting, given what they know about surgical uncertainty and thus the difficulty with offering meaningful reassurance to a very scared patient.

The surprise experienced by Wendy, when encountering this patient's panicky reluctance to separate from the student nurse and be handed on to her and other theatre staff, puts into focus the institutional expectation for patients to seamlessly transfer their trust from one nurse to the next nurse on the surgical journey. While there is a good skill-mix rationale for such fragmentation of caring relationships, this example perhaps illustrates how accountability and any resultant anxiety is curtailed by institutional processes which hand over patient responsibility.

In her work, Wendy uses this surprise as a spur to consider nurse-patient interaction and relationships. She notices the difference between how this patient uses her and the student nurse. Because of noticing her mixed, rivalrous emotional reactions to feeling pushed away and made emotionally redundant, Wendy focused on nursing this nurse–patient couple. This is achieved by establishing a cooperative and collaborative, rather than authoritarian and competitive, relationship with this student. In such a way, Wendy was able to nurse the couple so that she could take over the emotional caretaker role.

Commentary on 'Pre-operative anxiety'

Wendy argues that the relationship between the patient and student nurse serves an attachment-caretaker function. The student was able to provide that secure emotional base which enabled the patient to manage this anxiety-provoking transition. Wendy argues that nurses confuse attachment needs, the developmentally appropriate need to have available reliable people who can act as a secure base in anxious times, with psychological dependency (caricatured as an imaginary patient who displays regressive neediness, self-centredness and blames others). She suggests confusing attachment with dependency is not helpful to patients, as legitimate attachment needs are not met.

As Wendy identifies, the whole issue of appropriate emotional engagement by nurses with patients is fraught with institutional worry and unease, spawning social defence traditions, such as 'do not get involved'. It seems from the clinical illustrations used, emotionality in the care relationship is inevitable, when undertaking a caretaking role, such as nursing. There is always the potential of an emotional cost for the nurse. Social system defences inevitably evolve to manage the anxiety that such emotional engagement provokes. However, it is important to identify that the more rigid the defences are (for instance, depersonalisation of the patient into a medical condition only) the more energy they require to maintain, leaving less energy available for the work.

References

Jacques, E. (1955). 'Social systems as defence against persecutory and depressive anxiety.' In *New Directions in Psychoanalysis*, ed. Klein, M. London: Maresfield, pp. 49–63.

Klein, M. (1946). 'Notes on some schizoid mechanisms.' *International Journal of Psycho-Analysis* 27: 99–110.

Menzies, I. E. P. (1970). *The Functioning of Social Systems as a Defence against Anxiety. Centre for Applied Social Research*, London: Tavistock Institute of Health Relations. pp. 95–121.

Chapter 10
Joe's story[1]
Mary Paget

Introduction

It is probably fair to state that there are many occasions in nursing when the interactions that take place leave the nurses involved with a range of emotions, from unease, or anger, to a sense of despair. Those nurses may attempt to explain these feelings as being caused by stress, heavy workload, or a sense of having failed the patient, in some physical fashion. As Dartington (1993) suggests, the working life of nurses is generally dominated by practical necessity and it is rare that nurses give credit to their own emotions in the work that they do, even though those same nurses may recognise the emotional upheavals of their patients or their relatives, when facing illness or death.

Nurses are generally extremely tolerant of the wide range of behaviours that are exhibited by their patients. There are times though, when the behaviour or words of a client are seen as inexplicable, as they may run contrary to that which is expected. Nurses too hold general agreement of the appropriate way to behave when dealing with their patients and find themselves perplexed when they themselves behave or respond in ways that are unusual. Yet Freud (cited by Shapiro 1965, p.15) tells us that even the most bizarre behaviours and the strangest of symptoms can make sense. A number of psychodynamic theories have been proposed which attempt to explain such reactions in people. Although these theories are difficult to demonstrate empirically, they do offer a tentative means of understanding actions and

[1]This chapter is a revised version of the following article: Pullen, M.L. (2002). 'Joe's story: reflections on a difficult interaction between a nurse and a patient's wife.' International Journal of Palliative Nursing 8(10): 481–599.

relationships. Blumenfield and Thompson (1985) caution that it is also necessary to consider the special meaning that the illness has for the individual concerned, this meaning to be considered in the context of past experiences, individual personality and coping strategies.

In this chapter, I aim to analyse an incident encountered while in clinical practice, with regard to the psychological reactions to the disease and the psychological care that may have been required. The incident under scrutiny occurred some years ago, while I worked as a ward sister in an environment that cared for acutely ill people aged over sixty-five years. A patient was admitted to this area, who will be referred to as Joe D. During Joe's hospitalisation, a series of interactions occurred between nursing staff and Joe's wife (Mrs D) which led to open conflict between the parties and caused distress to all concerned. In an attempt to understand the prevailing influences on the participants, these interactions will be discussed with regard to specific psychodynamic theories relating to grief and the use of defence mechanisms (especially projection and projective identification).

Joe's story

Joe's story

Joe had a long history of heart disease, with multiple admissions to a variety of clinical areas for management of his cardiac failure. During previous admissions, a pattern had been established in which Joe was admitted to hospital in a very poor state, various medications would be given and gradually his condition would improve to a level which, although below his previous best, was sufficient to allow his discharge home into his wife's care.

During this admission, he had been given a variety of interventions and medications which had proved unsuccessful and it was determined that this time, Joe was unlikely to survive. However, it would appear that neither Joe nor his wife had been prepared for the insidious and ultimately terminal nature of heart disease. Instead, a sense of optimism and hope had been fostered that, although appropriate in the initial stages of the disease process, were now becoming unrealistic and unachievable in the face of Joe's impending death.

Joe and his wife were both Polish immigrants, who had lived in this country for many years. They had no sons or daughters, nor did they have any family in this country. Consequently, in the wake of Joe's illness, his wife had become his main caregiver, a role that she undertook devotedly. During Joe's stay in hospital, his wife remained present with him for much of the day, during which she undertook much of Joe's care, despite her own exhaustion from a long day that also included bus travel. Her exhaustion was exacerbated by the need to return home to launder Joe's clothes and make food for him to eat the following day. In addition to this, she cajoled him to eat or drink at frequent intervals, never resting herself, nor allowing Joe to rest either.

Into this background were introduced several new issues. The first was that medical interventions were currently not proving successful, Joe's symptoms of cardiac failure were not improving; indeed they were getting worse. He was acutely breathless, even at rest, and was exhausted by the least activity and movement. Conventional combinations of diuretic therapies were no longer proving effective, so Joe was incredibly oedematous, with leaking of serous fluid from his legs. It was impossible to change his position to any extent, as the effort left him acutely breathless and scared. Without movement, Joe became acutely uncomfortable. On the rare occasions that Joe became comfortable enough or relaxed enough to fall asleep, his wife would wake him up to try to make him eat or drink something.

At this point, faced with the hopeless nature of Joe's disease, both nursing and medical staff recognised that the focus of care had changed from a restorative aim towards palliative care. This was understood as the need to manage symptoms and to make preparation for death. Discussion ensued and both nurses and doctors agreed that, with the permission of his wife, Joe would be commenced on a device called a syringe driver pump, which would deliver small continuous doses of a combination of drugs, in an attempt to relieve his breathlessness and his fear. It was recognised that this might slightly shorten Joe's life, but this was balanced with the hope that his symptoms would be better relieved, improving his quality of life for the final few days of his life.

All this was explained to Joe's wife and she appeared to understand the main elements of the planned care and gave permission for the syringe driver to be commenced. This was also explained to Joe, but he appeared not to comprehend, as both hypoxia and language difficulties interfered with his capacity to understand. With everyone's agreement, the syringe driver was commenced, with a cocktail of diamorphine to relieve cardiac congestion and to relax Joe, a drug to improve breathing and a diuretic to reduce fluid overload. The cocktail and the mode of delivery appeared to work for Joe. He became less restless, less distressed by breathing difficulties and spent more time in sleep. When awake, he appeared more relaxed and was able to communicate a few sentences with less interference from breathing problems.

The following day, Joe's wife came into the nurses' office, claiming that: 'You are trying to murder my husband!' She was shaking and white with anger and would not even attempt to listen to any of the questions, or explanations posed by the nursing staff, myself included. Eventually, it emerged that she believed that because Joe was sleeping for much of the time, and was unable to eat and drink with the same frequency she had previously insisted upon, this meant that he would 'starve' and that it was 'your fault'.

Everyone was puzzled by this attitude; after all, Joe was dying and his wife apparently understood this fact. Food and drink had been problematic to him for some time, as his breathing problems interfered with chewing and swallowing. In fact, many of the ward staff had voiced concern that Joe's wife had not recognised his need to rest and had constantly interrupted any rest by making him eat or drink. A number of nurses had voiced their satisfaction at the rest that Joe was now getting and had commented on his apparent peacefulness. If he were now to die, at least it would be a 'good' death; that is a death unaccompanied by pain, fear or the distress accompanying his inability to breathe.

I tried to explain these observations to Joe's wife. At this point she rounded on me and accused me personally of trying to murder her husband: 'You forced him to have the syringe driver and now it is killing him!' While it was true that the previous day I had been instrumental in discussing the need for an alternative route to deliver the medication and actively involved in gaining consent for this, it was clearly not my sole decision to proceed with this form of treatment. I felt affronted and shocked that such an accusation had been made. At this point, I recognised that I could not deal with Mrs D alone, so asked my nurse manager to assist and intervene.

The outcome was that Mrs D would not be reconciled to her husband's impending death. She continued to believe that the syringe driver was instrumental in killing him and subsequently, the syringe driver was discontinued. Joe died several days later in acute distress.

Discussion

Mr and Mrs D were Jews in Poland at the time of the war. As a young married couple, they were fortunate to escape to Britain at a time when Nazi pogroms against Jews were becoming commonplace in Poland. However, the family members that remained in Poland were not so lucky; they were incarcerated in concentration camps where they ultimately died. I know little about how individual family members died, other than Joe making brief reference to this on a previous admission to hospital. There has been sufficient subsequent information about concentration camps to assume that they did not die comfortably.

Karon and Widener (1995) suggest that experiences, memories and feelings can be repressed into the unconscious if they are too frightening or guilt-provoking to deal with consciously. Freud (cited by Bongar and Beutler, 1995, pp. 26–7) described a number of defence mechanisms that are essential to normal functioning and serve to keep painful or distressing feelings at a manageable level. Heyse-Moore (2007) also suggests that these feelings can resurface when one is close to death. It may be reasonable to assume that Mrs D felt some degree of guilt at leaving her family behind, even though she may not have been able to anticipate the outcome. There may be an analogy drawn with her behaviour while Joe was in hospital. She stayed with him from early in the morning until late at night, despite her own exhaustion. It is possible that unconsciously, Mrs D was afraid to leave him; after all, the last time she left loved ones behind, they died in awful circumstances.

Mr and Mrs D did not have any children and it appeared that they devoted their lives to each other, evidenced by her devoted care for her husband. She anticipated and provided for his every need; Joe had only to ask for something and it was provided. Even in hospital, she helped him with feeding, washing, dressing and even toileting, allowing the nurses to carry out only procedures that she was unfamiliar with.

Bowlby (1969) considers that during each phase of our lives, we make strong emotional bonds to a few special individuals. It is clear that Mr and Mrs D's relationship typified such bonding. Bowlby (1969) also suggests that the breaking of these bonds, through involuntary separation and/or death is a time of extreme anxiety and distress. It is likely that in the light of their shared experiences as a young married couple, as well as their lack of children, the news of Joe's closeness to death would bring unbearable stress, fear and pain to Mrs D.

It is perhaps less surprising then that Mrs D responded with anger. Blumenfield and Thompson (1985) state that becoming angry is a common way of dealing with fear; an unbearable feeling is transformed into one that is easier and more comfortable to express. Bowlby and Murray Parkes (1970) suggest that anger is a biological survival response to temporary separation; the reproaches made after reunion strengthen bonds and aim to make future separations less likely.

Kübler-Ross (1970) affirms that anger is one of the key emotions experienced by those who are receiving news about an impending death. Rather than being inappropriate, anger should be expected. Parkes (1975, p. 209) later commented that 'the greater the grief the greater the inclination to avoid it', suggesting that anger can be a defence against grief. For Mrs D, it is likely that her grief was immense, not just from the impending loss of Joe, but also because Joe's death would also result in the loss of her remaining family. Her world was about to fall apart.

Mrs D was extremely angry, this anger may have been directed unconsciously at Joe, as he was about to leave her permanently but Mrs D probably could not express this anger to Joe. After all Joe was the one who was dying, so it seems plausible to suggest that her anger was displaced from Joe and targeted at and expressed to a more suitable recipient, the nurse in charge of the ward where her husband was dying.

Additionally, Joe was about to leave her completely alone, with no one else to turn to. Bowlby (1969) argued that one of the most disturbing feelings aroused by loss is the fear of abandonment. Mrs D appeared to be working exceptionally hard to ensure that the ties between her and Joe remained strong, constantly reinforcing these ties with endearments and tender care. There was likely to be no substitute for the loss of Joe, so it became desirable, even essential that Joe survive.

In this case, husband and wife could be seen as a closely functioning unit. It is difficult to conceive of any situation where this unit is split into its two respective halves, one of which must continue to function in the absence of the other. Such anticipation may have led Mrs D to deny Joe's impending death, as a defence against a sense of disintegration, thereby accounting for her difficulty in acknowledging the changing nature of their relationship.

Unlike many patients' relatives who appear relieved to either shed or share the burden of care once a patient is admitted to a hospital, Mrs D remained actively involved in Joe's care throughout his stay. This apparent need to care was expressed through practical actions and presence, as Mrs D was available whenever Joe needed her and indeed Joe frequently checked that she was present. This is congruent with Bowlby's (1969) reminder that in illness we seek the presence of those we know and trust, as to be detached from a particular caretaker is a situation that is instinctively fraught with danger.

Judd (1989) suggests that when one is involved with the dying, one may have conscious feelings of guilt for having 'failed' the patient and a sense of responsibility for the death. These are often mixed with unconscious feelings of hatred towards loved ones that form a normal part of early development. Gomez (1997) explains the origins of such feelings, using Winnicott's stance on the development of the infant's early self. She suggests that immediately after birth, the mother becomes near-obsessed with her new baby (termed primary maternal preoccupation), fostering an illusion of oneness with the baby that makes the baby feel secure and powerful. As the mother begins to take up her own separate life again, this preoccupation naturally wanes, the infant gradually realises that mother is not under its control, that its own powers are limited and it is indeed a separate entity. For the infant this is accompanied by feelings of frustration, disillusionment and sometimes hatred. Guilt and a wish to repair the imagined damage caused by hateful feelings are a consequence. Patients who do not respond to curative treatment can be felt to thwart the best reparative efforts of doctors, nurses and relatives, leaving all carers exposed to feelings of hatred and guilt which are not easy to alleviate.

When such disillusioning experiences are too intense or too frequent for the baby to cope with, a range of anxieties may follow that Winnicott (1988) describes as 'going to pieces'; 'having no relation to the body'; 'having no orientation in the world' and a feeling of 'complete isolation' with little means of communication. Winnicott also suggests that these anxieties can resurface in later life, at times of difficulty.

It is possible to imagine that these may have been some of the emotions that Joe was experiencing. As his world grew smaller, becoming restricted only to a hospital bay and the presence of his wife and his nurses, Joe may have lost his sense of where he belonged in the world. Similarly, as his body was causing him immense pain and discomfort, no longer obeying his commands, he may have lost his sense of relationship to his body. His breathing difficulties could have provoked feelings of isolation and panic, with the added frustration of having to rely on someone else to interpret his needs.

Winnicott suggests that the mother protects the infant from these experiences, presenting the world to the infant in manageable doses and through 'holding', a process of protecting the infant from too many unpleasant experiences and empathising with and soothing the infant when such experiences occur. The mother is able to do this through her attunement to the infant's needs and emotions. It is possible that Mrs D was acting as a mother figure might, adapting herself to the needs of her charge and protecting him from those anxieties and stressors he was too sick to deal with.

Klein (1932, cited by Money-Kyrle, 1984) explains this 'attunement' in terms of infant development; the infant has little sense of time, very little language with which to communicate and his main sensations will relate to being mothered: held, fed, bathed and talked to, but also in relation to being hungry, in pain, anxious or left alone. In order to deal with these feelings, the infant develops a defence mechanism which involves isolating these 'good' and 'bad' sensations from itself and projecting them into a suitable external object, usually the mother. This projection of feelings is achieved through non-verbal communication, which the mother picks up on and may experience within herself.

In a similar way, Mrs D was clearly able to anticipate Joe's needs without him needing to vocalise them and to carry out his care in ways that Joe was both comfortable and familiar with. This may tentatively explain some of the conflict that existed between Mrs D and the nursing staff. After all, Mrs D was effectively carrying out most of the role traditionally carried out by nurses. Nursing, according to Peplau (1988) is about anticipating and meeting the needs of those who are sick, through the use of a therapeutic relationship. A part of this role often involves the 'holding' of patients' emotions, as well as allowing them to be expressed in a way that is meaningful and therapeutic. Many nurses, including myself, expressed resentment of Mrs D's actions in caring for Joe, as that caring eroded many aspects of their own role. Certainly, I recall feeling frustration and anger that it seemed impossible to 'get close' to Joe because of the continual presence of his wife, as well as a sense that I was not allowed to fulfil my caring role effectively and without interference.

Nurses do not become immune to the anxieties that the prospective death of a patient will bring. Rather, nurses cope with this by trying to be useful to the dying person, to relieve symptoms and distress and to provide a level of care that assuages our feelings. Mrs D deprived me of this coping strategy. It is possible that this generated a sense of rivalry, fostering my own resentment and leaving me feeling useless in Joe's care.

It is also possible that the feelings that I experienced were directly related to the emotions being experienced by Mrs D, that she may have been projecting into me. Mrs D may have been experiencing frustration that her husband was not getting any better, anger with him as he was about to leave her and anger at the nurses for introducing the issue of Joe's dying and destroying her hopes of his recovery. She also could have felt that the nurses were interfering in her caring role, separating her from Joe when they needed each other.

One role that Mrs D undertook was her constant feeding of Joe. Feeding is considered to be a nurturing task (Winnicott, 1988), one that comforts, develops and nourishes. It is also necessary for life. Indeed the act of feeding another is perhaps one of the most fundamental offerings that one human can make to another. This may partly explain Mrs D's apparent need to wake Joe frequently in order to insist on his taking food and drink. Another explanation may relate to Joe and Mrs D's wartime experiences as Jews in Poland. It is well documented that many Jews were 'ghettoised', this process being associated with deprivation and starvation. In this context, food would become so important that not one mouthful would be wasted, to waste food would be to perish.

Feeding is also very intimate. One has only to reflect on the content of some films where feeding a partner is a precursor to further intimacy. Clearly such intimacy was impossible, given Joe's very sick condition, yet traces of that intimacy could perhaps be read into her act of feeding him. However, this action clearly became inappropriate the sicker Joe became. He was too breathless to take more than a few sips of fluid or mouthfuls of food, yet Mrs D continually prompted him to eat and drink. This led to Joe becoming more and more exhausted and less inclined to take any oral sustenance, yet Mrs D persisted. On the occasions when nurses gently suggested that Joe could benefit from a rest, she became affronted and chose to ignore such suggestions. Perhaps Mrs D simply could not acknowledge the truth of Joe's dying condition. By adopting such a maternal role, which is essentially about nurturing and developing, she may have been unconsciously attempting to defy the odds and make him well again.

An alternative explanation for Mrs D's persistence in feeding Joe is based on Caplan's (1961) suggestion that major life stresses disrupt the customary modes of behaviour of the people concerned. When the strain exceeds a certain threshold of severity, individuals become overwhelmed by it and find themselves persevering in activities which may have been helpful in the past but which are inappropriate to the present situation. In such circumstances, old assumptions and behaviours may be adhered to rigidly. For Mrs D, feeding Joe would have been an activity which in the past would have helped him recover from his many hospital admissions and helped protect herself from the anxiety of Joe's illness.

Similarly, allowing Joe to sleep may have been too close to the idea of 'going for the long sleep' or even of 'being put to sleep', creating feelings of great distress that had to be repressed into the unconscious. On a symbolic level, not allowing Joe to sleep could be construed as keeping him alive. When she eventually left for the night, it was always accompanied by promises of special food treats that she would bring the following day, as well as 'nice, clean pyjamas'. It was almost as though she tacitly made him promise to stay alive overnight, so that he could look forward to and experience the treats she would bring.

Mrs D, it seems, was desperately attempting to keep her husband alive, yet this was presented in a way that appeared almost inhumane to the nurses, who were anticipating his death. Mrs D's desire to keep him alive was in direct contrast and in conflict with the desire of the nurses to facilitate a peaceful death.

Nurses too, tend to have a picture of an ideal death. This ideal is represented by peaceful sleep, by being allowed to drift off comfortably into death, allowing only measures that promote comfort rather than a longer life, without futile, distressing attempts to prolong life. So although all parties clearly wanted the best for Joe, the 'best' for the participants seemed to differ completely.

Mrs D appeared to be very distrustful of any nursing interventions. For example, whenever new medications were introduced, she closely interrogated the nurses about their purpose and associated side-effects. She closely monitored the times when medications should be given and was quick to comment, should those medications be a few minutes late or early. When it was finally suggested to her that a 'syringe driver' infusion pump be started to provide the best means of administering Joe's medication, this too was greeted with numerous questions and a degree of suspicion.

Later on, when Joe appeared more relaxed and sleepy as his symptoms became better controlled, Mrs D may have interpreted this as confirmation that the institution was indeed trying to kill her husband. Such a persecutory belief was expressed vividly through her accusation that I was trying to 'murder' her husband.

It is possible to feel some considerable empathy for the dilemma Mrs D must have found herself in. On the one hand, she didn't really trust anyone from the institution, yet the institution was her only means of keeping her husband alive. She must have felt emotionally torn, with such conflicting desires. Yet her behaviour made it difficult for me to express any feelings of empathy towards her. Instead, I felt extremely hurt, disbelieving, angry and threatened.

It is also worth considering how this style of functioning could be reflected in the behaviour of the nurses. While most nurses are comfortable with limited involvement of carers in the hospital environment, it is likely that the nurses had difficulty accepting the extent to which Mrs D wished to provide care, unfairly looking at any flaws in her ability to care as evidence that they, the nurses, would do a better job. In addition, Mrs D's multiple questions about treatment plans felt threatening, leading to suspicion and distrust about Mrs D's motives in asking those questions.

As stated earlier, projection is an unconscious process where emotions are split off from one person and believed to belong to another person, who may well be a good recipient for these emotions (for example: an angry person becomes a good recipient of other people's angry projections). It is a way of trying to cope with anxieties and stresses and of making a link to another person. Projective identification is a more extreme form of projection, where the recipient may feel some form of the emotion being projected, as if it were actually being inserted into him/her. Symington (1986) suggests that when this occurs, the recipient feels what the ego of the other feels.

Earlier, when describing this situation, I stated that I felt 'affronted' by Mrs D's accusations that I was trying to kill Joe. In analysing this, I think that the term 'affronted' probably does not come close to the emotions that I felt at the time. In retrospect, I think better words would be panicky, bewildered, misunderstood and scared.

This suggests that my own emotions at the time could have been a response to Mrs D's emotions, which if projected into me, allowed her to temporarily disown the pain of experiencing those emotions herself, as well as communicating the importance of these feelings to me. It is possible that, had I interpreted my own feelings in this way, I would have been more able to contain my feelings and as a result would have been better able to help Mrs D with hers. As it was, the feelings aroused in me by such a confrontation were so strong, that I felt I could no longer deal with Mrs D and called for assistance from a more senior nurse.

It is also worth considering whether some of the feelings of the nursing staff were being projected into Mrs D. Commencing a syringe driver on terminally ill patients is always a treatment that is delivered after much debate and consultation with staff. It is well known that some patients, when relieved from the distress of their symptoms, will actually regain some of their strength and appear to rally for some time. Others relax and are able to die quietly and peacefully. The problem for nurses is that it is rarely possible to judge in advance which outcome will occur, consequently many dread being the person to set up the infusion, especially where opiate drugs are used. There is a strong association between narcotic use and respiratory depression; many nurses are therefore concerned about delivering such drugs to patients with breathing difficulties. Tarzian (2000) reports that there is considerable research demonstrating their effectiveness and that giving an overdose to such a patient is unlikely because their narcotic tolerance levels are high. Even so, nurses are justifiably concerned that their actions are correctly interpreted. There is the moral principle of double effect. This claims that it is not morally wrong to administer drugs that may shorten a patient's life as long as those drugs are prescribed with the intent of alleviating symptoms, rather than deliberately shortening life. Tarzian summarised it as:

> ... if you're going to die of respiratory arrest, is it the respiratory arrest because your lungs finally gave out or is the respiratory arrest because you had a little too much morphine? You know, it almost doesn't matter at that point. (Tarzian, 2000, p. 141)

Despite this, it remains a concern of most nurses to walk this fine line. Tarzian referred to palliative care as 'fine-tuning' the symptoms and process of dying, but recognises the complexity of such actions. In a busy medical ward, there is always concern that the fine-tuning may not be supervised closely enough.

Mrs D may have had an awareness of our doubts and anxieties. It would be natural then for her to question the staff about the use and effects of such an infusion. Sensing such doubt may have made her more convinced that we were unsure of the outcome and were perhaps experimenting on her husband, using syringes and drugs. This too may have found echoes in her past, resulting in her outburst to me: 'You are killing him, you are murdering my Joe!' This statement poignantly demonstrates some of the anguish she must have been feeling at that time; her body language too indicated the depth of her distress, as she was white and shaking. I interpreted this at the time as being in a state of extreme anger, but in retrospect, it is plausible to suggest that her reaction may have been one of extreme distress due to fear.

It is also true that Mrs D touched upon my own vulnerabilities. As a nurse, I was fully aware of the legal and ethical debate surrounding the use of opiate medications in terminally ill patients and was always able to use these arguments to justify, consciously, my own participation in such activities. However, at the same time, I was also aware that I could be hastening the death of another being. I think it likely that Mrs D's accusation brought this uncomfortable truth to the surface. This grain of truth was difficult to deal with as it linked directly to my own guilt and conflict about my actions, the sense that my actions might be maleficent rather than beneficent. It is possible that I projected these feelings into Mrs D, that her accusation resonated with an inner accusing voice of my own.

As stated earlier, my emotions were also of fear, anger, hurt and disbelief. Certainly, in this interaction, I clearly felt out of my depth and contacted a senior nurse to intervene. I wonder if my own actions in calling for another individual to help with this situation were an example of adopting a primitive defence mechanism. It could be that the anxiety induced by the accusation led me into the regressive action of turning to 'mother' to deal with the situation, much as a child would turn to its mother for help with a situation beyond its control.

Fortunately, the senior nurse made herself available immediately and took Mrs D aside for some time to calm down and to discuss the issues. Mrs D did calm down eventually, but this was based on the promise that the syringe driver would be discontinued forthwith. My own feelings about this were mixed. I could understand the decision, given the nature of the accusations made, but felt disappointed that it was likely that Joe would now die in a ghastly fashion, with severe breathing distress and its associated feelings of panic and fright.

Mrs D did not become any easier to deal with however. It is possible that discontinuing the infusion may have reinforced and confirmed her conviction that we were indeed killing her husband. She became even more vigilant and rarely left his side, even for her own needs. The effect on the nursing staff in general is hard to capture, but I recall feeling it necessary to handle Mrs D with 'kid gloves', being careful of every word uttered, so that it was not misinterpreted. I regret that my care of Joe probably suffered, as it was easier to stay away and allow

Mrs D to deliver care, rather than face her questions and implicit accusations (and rather than face my own guilty feelings?). Where medications were concerned, although it was usual practice for two nurses to prepare and check all drugs, these were now prepared and checked at the bedside in front of Mrs D. I practised defensively and with a feeling of dread. Joe died some days later, with very little symptom relief. I would not wish that death on anyone.

I do not believe that I was the only nurse who found this situation stressful. Butterworth (1992) coined the phrase 'Tea break/Tear break', to describe the informal mechanisms that nurses utilise in order to relieve their stress or distress. Although at the time, few tears were actually spilt, many nurses used such tea breaks to express their feelings and to receive support from each other. Although informal, it is possible that this ad hoc support system helped those nurses involved in Joe's care to temporarily regain some emotional equilibrium, sufficient to enable them to continue to deliver care. It is also possible that the lack of structured discussion led to a situation where the 'problem' of Mrs D and Joe was magnified. Although informal discussion may have helped the nurses to cope with the trauma of Joe's dying, there was little shared understanding or insight into the behaviour of Mrs D. This meant that the nurses were unlikely to be able to help her in any meaningful way.

Certainly, at the time of this incident, I would have welcomed some form of emotional support. Mrs D's accusation that I was murdering her husband wounded me deeply and following her accusation, I was fearful that when Joe eventually died, I would be held accountable for his death and punished accordingly. As my senior nurse had become involved, I was also afraid that this would act as a 'black mark' against my professional abilities. Had I had the opportunity to explore these issues with a trusted supervisor, it is likely that my feelings would have been better clarified. After all, acknowledging one's feelings is often the first step towards dealing with stress. My subsequent care of Joe may have been to a better standard, but as it was my fears and emotions kept me away from Joe's bedside and prevented me from delivering effective care.

Conclusion

Hospitals are places that are full of emotions. When things go well a nurse may be showered with praise, affection and gratitude. However, when health fails, that same nurse may be the recipient of the frustrations and resentments of their clients. According to Menzies Lyth (1988) hospitals are places where nurses in particular must allow the projection of feelings such as depression or anxiety into them. This adds to the nurse's own intense anxieties and leaves her/him at risk of 'being flooded by intense and unmanageable anxiety' (Menzies Lyth, 1988, p. 50).

This one episode of patient care has indicated some of the complexities of the nurse–patient–relative relationship; most nurses in clinical practice have to deal with such complexities on a daily basis. Given the emotional content of such interactions, it is unsurprising that many nurses feel physically and emotionally drained at the end of a span of duty. If this persists over time, such emotional distress can lead to the condition known as 'burnout' and the loss of nurses from the profession.

Barber (1993) considers that the nursing profession has developed a culture where nurses' fears are not acknowledged, their worries are not worked through and their vulnerabilities are hidden, often from themselves. Such feelings are often repressed, but along the way, nurses can lose their sensitivity when dealing with patients. In just such a fashion, my own fears were not really addressed and the nursing care that I was able to deliver to Joe suffered as a result. This too has been a source of unresolved guilt and concern to me over the years. In some ways, the writing of this chapter has proved cathartic, allowing me to both analyse my actions and to absolve myself of many of the guilty feelings that I have carried. Had a form of clinical supervision been available at the time of the incident, I too may have enjoyed the benefits of a therapeutic relationship and been able to assist other nurses in similar ways.

I don't know to what extent I could have helped Mrs D. After all, she was a product of her past experiences and her coping mechanisms were already well established. However, in this situation her coping mechanisms were evidently not enough. It is possible that had I been helped to recognise my own emotional response to the situation, as well as having the opportunity to explore possible reasons for Mrs D's emotional outburst and general behaviour, I may have been better able to contain her feelings and provide her with support. At the very least, I may have better understood her feelings and been less afraid to care for Joe. The outcome for Joe may have been different.

The commentary for this chapter has been combined with that for the next chapter and therefore appears following Chapter 11.

References

Barber, P. (1993). 'Developing the "person" of the professional carer.' In *Nursing Practice and Health Care*, eds. S.M. Hinchliff, S.E. Norman, and J.E. Schober, 2nd edn. London: Edward Arnold, pp. 344–73.

Bongar, B. and Beutler, L.E. (1995). *Comprehensive Textbook of Psychotherapy.* New York: Oxford University Press.

Bowlby, J. (1969). 'Affectional bonds: their nature and origin.' In *Progress in Mental Health; Proceedings of the Seventh International Congress on Mental Health*, ed. H. Freeman. London: J. and A. Churchill, pp. 319—27.

Bowlby, J. and Murray Parkes, C. (1970). 'Separation and loss within the family.' In *The Child in his Family. Vol 1. International Yearbook of Child Psychiatry and Allied Professions*, eds. E.J. Anthony and C. Koupernik. New York: Wiley, pp. 197–216.

Blumenfield, M. and Thompson, T.L. (1985). 'The psychological reactions to illness.' In *Understanding Human Behaviour in Health and Illness*, R.C. Simons, 3rd edn. London: Williams and Wilkins, pp. 48–59.

Butterworth, T. (1992). 'Clinical supervision as an emerging idea in nursing.' In *Clinical Supervision and Mentorship in Nursing*, eds. T. Butterworth and J. Faugier. London: Chapman and Hall, pp. 3–18.

Caplan, G. (1961). *An Approach to Community Mental Health.* New York: Grunne and Stratton.

Dartington, A. (1993). 'Where angels fear to tread. Idealism, despondency and inhibition in thought in hospital nursing.' *Winnicott Studies* **7**: 21–41.

Gomez, L. (1997). *An Introduction to Object Relations.* London: Free Association Books.

Heyse-Moore, L. (2007). 'Dying to talk.' *Therapy Today* **18** (5) June: 11–14.

Judd, D. (1989). *Give Sorrow Words.* London: Free Association Books.

Karon, B.P. and Widener, A.J. (1995). 'Psychodynamic therapies in historical perspective.' In *Comprehensive Textbook of Psychotherapy*, B. Bongar and L.E. Beutler. New York: Oxford University Press.

Kübler-Ross, E. (1970). *On Death and Dying.* London: Tavistock.

Menzies Lyth, I. (1988). *Containing Anxiety in Institutions: Selected Essays*, Vol. I. London: Free Association Books.

Money-Kyrle, R. ed. (1984). *The Writings of Melanie Klein*, Vol. 2. New York: Free Press.

Parkes, C.M. (1975). 'Psycho-social transitions: comparison between reactions to loss of a limb and loss of a spouse.' *British Journal of Psychiatry* **127**: 204–10.

Peplau, H. (1988). *Interpersonal Relations in Nursing*. New York: Putnam.

Shapiro, D. (1965). *Neurotic Styles*. New York: Basic Books Inc.

Symington, N. (1986). *The Analytic Experience*. London: Free Association Books.

Tarzian, A.J. (2000). 'Caring for dying patients who have air hunger.' *Journal of Nursing Scholarship* **32**(2): 137–43.

Winnicott, D.W. (1988). 'Breast feeding as communication.' In *Babies and Their Mothers*. London: Free Association Books, pp. 23–49.

Chapter 11

Thoughts on the impact of a suicide
Alyson Charnock

Introduction

This chapter will attempt to interpret a care scenario, from the author's perspective, in relation to the psychodynamic theories of counter-transference and projective identification. The second part of the chapter will introduce the theory to analyse the scenario, to make sense of the interactive processes between the main characters in the event. The theories of counter-transference and projective identification are defined and the links between them explored. These theories come from psychoanalysis but an attempt is made here to apply them to the world of nursing. The chapter concludes with a short critical discussion regarding the nature of the analysis. The main focus is one of interpretation and application of theory to practice, so no attempt will be made to critically evaluate one theory over another.

There now follows a narrative which describes the events of a seven-day period occurring during an episode of care. I was then an experienced staff nurse working in a very busy acute admission area in an urban Psychiatric Unit. The person being cared for was a twenty-three-year-old man, diagnosed some time previously as suffering from schizophrenia, the central object of the story however, is not the patient, but the patient's mother, Mrs Smith, the main carer in this particular situation.

The scenario

The scenario

It was late morning on a normal Thursday on an acute psychiatric ward. There were twenty-four patients and the ward was full to overflowing with patients, visitors, doctors and occupational therapists. I was in charge of the shift that day and felt fine, fully in control of what was going on, aware of what was left to do before the afternoon shift came on duty. My one concern amidst the chaos was John, a young schizophrenic who had become increasingly withdrawn as the week progressed. The night before, I had taken the decision to place John on the highest level of clinical observation, one-to-one nursing, which was to be reviewed by the Medical Officer in charge of John's care that morning. On the doctor's arrival, I expressed my concern for John and asked if he could be seen as a matter of priority. The doctor invited John to the interview room but declined a nurse escort when his nurse got up to go with them. I asked the doctor to ring the office when the interview was over, as the room was in another part of the ward. The ward had a CCTV system with an alarm, which sounded if someone opened the main door. A little while after the doctor had left, the alarm sounded and John was seen running down the stairs.

John had a long history of persecutory delusions and had been admitted several times in a short space of time, always being identified as a risk to himself and, therefore, usually admitted under a section of the Mental Health Act. Nurses were very shortly seen on the CCTV link in the ward office running down the stairs after John, in an attempt to bring him back. John could not be found in the grounds so the police were contacted, the 'absent without leave' procedure initiated and his parents informed.

John's parents (Mr and Mrs Smith) were both in their sixties, wealthy, respected people in their community who were childless until they adopted John as a toddler. John was their life. He was particularly close to his mother who visited at least twice a day. It was always hoped John would take over the family business, even when he was diagnosed, there was still hope that he would recover sufficiently to be able to run the firm effectively. No amount of explaining and education would change their minds; John may have been ill but to them, he was not severely ill and he would be cured of his illness to live the life they had prepared for him.

I rang John's mother to tell her he had left the ward, and the circumstances surrounding his departure; his parents arrived on the ward very soon afterwards. John's mother was extremely upset, but very confident that I would locate John and bring him back, as if I was the one who would physically be out looking for John. She outwardly appeared very cool and calm but underneath the surface something was brewing, there was more than a hint of fear in her voice.

I explained the 'absent without leave' procedure, that the police had received a report about John, his clothing, height, build etc. and that they would patrol the area around the hospital and his home that day and generally keep a lookout for anyone that matched his description. She seemed not to hear this, but expressed fear for his safety, fear that he was lost, that he was afraid. She constantly repeated that I would make everything all right, that I had done so on previous admissions and I would do so again. This was not the first time that I had experienced patients absconding from the ward. It was a regular occurrence on this busy admission unit and was accepted as being part of the job. Patients ran away and got brought back, much more rarely a patient would be found dead, but it happened and it had happened to me before.

As soon as John's mother left the office, I began to experience a rising sense of panic and helplessness and a sense of futility with the whole situation. I suspected that John would kill himself and I knew that I could do nothing to prevent it. I felt afraid that he would die, afraid that I had done something wrong. I had not felt like this in connection with a patient before. John's mother had sat herself in the lounge, sitting opposite the door where she could see me at the desk. It didn't seem appropriate to close the door, or to ask her to leave as she was waiting for her husband to arrive and for any news which she said she thought would come soon after her arrival.

The shift passed and there was no news, but John's mother did not move. The office door was eventually closed for the hand-over. Sometime later, I came out of the office to go home and stopped to talk to her. She was still insisting that I could make things better, that things would be all right. I still felt extremely panicked about the whole situation and I must have looked equally worried and upset. I was very uncomfortable talking to John's mother, very afraid that she would lose her son but couldn't tell her so. Externally she looked very calm, very in control, when telling me that she would leave when I did. Initially, she seemed almost surprised that I would be going home. She didn't say it but I felt she thought that I should stay until everything was sorted out, until John came back. On getting home, I had an urge to ring the

Nurses and their patients

ward, to ask how things were going, and I did. I never, ever do this. I have never needed to, until this event. It didn't make me feel any better. I had the urge to ring again before I went to bed but didn't. I am usually able to leave things in work, to take my 'nursing hat' off, but I couldn't. The sense of panic, fear, hopelessness and frustration stayed with me over the next few days and I was having difficulty sleeping, doing, thinking about anything other than John and his probable fate.

John's mother was a regular visitor to the ward over this period. She would sit with his things and say nothing to anyone except me. She did ask for my home phone number once, but this was denied her, so she just sat and waited for me to come on duty without speaking to anyone. Her verbal statements of confidence in me continued, up until five days later when we got the call to say that John had been found.

John was found on a local beach. He had drowned, but the pathologist later said that he had only been in the sea for around twenty-four hours; damage to his body was limited. This meant he had been staying somewhere for around four days prior to his eventual suicide. The call came during an afternoon shift; I was in charge of the shift and took the call, informed John's parents (who were on the ward) and went to identify the body, as his parents had declined the task. My relationship with John's mother changed as soon as I told her what had happened. She withdrew totally, became distant and cool with me. She simply said 'Thank you' and turned away. It may have been easier if she had been angry, or shouted at me, told me I was bad or wrong and should have done something else. I felt mortally wounded, I was extremely sad, it was physically painful.

After the shift I continued to feel a sense of extreme sadness, I felt a sense of loss, of failure and this went on for a period of days. I can feel it even now, when I think about that period in time, although time helped the pain. I was debriefed by the senior nurse, basically a pat on the head and an emotional sticking plaster administered with a 'there, there, it's all right' mentality.

I still see John's mother around town, usually on the weekends. She looks at me as if I am not there, not even a glance, but I still feel the pain, the hate as she walks past. If I see her coming, I will cross the street; the physical distance makes the feelings easier to bear.

Thoughts on the impact of a suicide

Theoretical overview

Theoretical overview

Counter-transference

Conceptions of counter-transference have ranged on a continuum from a narrow definition: a person's reaction to another's transference, to a blanket statement: the totality of the analyst's reaction to his/her patient (Schroder, 1985). Broadly speaking, counter-transference in the nurse–patient relationship has been described as thoughts and feelings experienced by the nurse which are relevant to the patient's internal world and which may be used by the nurse to understand the meaning of their patients' communications, to help rather than hinder treatment (Bateman and Holmes, 1995). Winnicott (1947) suggests that counter-transference is something that should be exploited by the practitioner, for example to feel hate, when it has been projected into you and evoked by the patient, is part of the practitioner's proper responsiveness. When the patient seeks the practitioner's hate, the practitioner must be able to feel it, to bear it without retaliating, thereby containing it, otherwise there is a possibility that feelings of mutual hostility may be enacted and the therapeutic value lost, through lack of understanding.

Schroder (1985) suggests that counter-transference should be assumed when the nurse has strong emotional reactions that are not normally experienced, for example, when it is necessary to ask other professionals about a particular patient or when normal practice boundaries are extended. For instance, the nurse may become preoccupied with the patient to an unusual degree when away from the patient and/or feel recurrent anxiety, unease or guilt related to the patient (Langs, 1974, cited by O'Kelly, 1998). As counter-transference is an intense response, it may also be manifested in the form of physical symptoms which are often identified with stress. Sweating, jaw clenching, tightening of abdominal or shoulder muscles were recognised as symptoms by which nurses could be more aware of counter-transference responses (O'Kelly, 1998).

Projective identification

The term 'projective identification' was introduced into psycho-analysis by Melanie Klein (1946, cited by Segal 1973) to describe specific interpersonal processes, where parts of the psyche, namely 'bad' feelings, are projected into the good breast. Put simply, it refers to a psychological process in which one person projects a thought, belief or emotion into a second person. Then there is another action in which the second person is changed by the projection and begins to behave as though he or she is in fact actually characterised by those thoughts or beliefs that have been projected. Klein (1946, cited by Segal, 1973) referred to phantasised or internal representations of actual relationships which are initiated to protect the person from internal destruction and to protect the 'good' feelings; 'bad' feelings are then hopefully modified by the recipient and re-introjected by the projector. Various parts of the self may be projected, with various aims: bad parts of the self may be projected in order to get rid of them, as well as to attack and destroy. Good parts may be projected to avoid separation or to keep them safe from bad things inside. Klein uses the 'ph' in phantasy, as opposed to fantasy to emphasise that this is an unconscious process. Hinshelwood (1991) suggests that as well as being the most fruitful Kleinian concept it is also the most confusing one. In further elaborations of the concept, it was seen as an important element of normal ego and personality development.

Segal (1973) provides a definition of projective identification as a defence mechanism, suggesting that it occurs when unacceptable parts of the self are split off and put into an external object that then carries this part for the person. Identification is maintained with the split off part so that the relationship can be maintained with that part of the self. The recipient of the split off part takes on a particular role that is thrust upon them, so those involved in projective identification, partially and temporarily share a sense of identity. The recipient experiences a degree or strength of feeling that is surprising, but though an exaggeration, is still his or hers.

Hughes and Pengelly (1997) give a more simplified definition of the unconscious process of projective identification, highlighting two distinct stages: the first being to get rid of difficult feelings that, at the time, cannot be tolerated; the second being to communicate the importance of the feelings by getting another person to experience them, in the hope that this second person will be better able to bear the feelings and give meaning to them.

There is a process of the projection finding a home and

unconscious collusion to work with the split-off part by the person receiving the projection. The recipient may find him/herself forced by the projector to feel the projector's own aggressive qualities and impulses which are otherwise alien to him. He may feel strange and uncomfortable and may resent what is happening, but in the face of the projector's position it may be doubly difficult to resist the feelings steadily forced into him.

Bion (1962) formulated a model of the container (nurse/analyst) and the contained (the projected emotions) which explicitly linked projective identification with normal developmental processes and which relates to the idea of normal counter-transference, which occurs constructively between analyst and client. One implication of Bion's container/contained model is that it permits the receiver of the evacuated experiences to formulate them as experiences of himself. Bion (1962), who also used the term 'passion' in relation to emotionality in the link between two minds, recommends that one does not listen to the patient, one listens to oneself listening to the patient. The container is believed to have immediate access to his own experiences, that is, he is believed to be capable of dealing with the patient's experiences as his own. These experiences Bion calls 'the contained' and their importance lies in their intensity and the challenge they present to the recipient to think about them rather than to react to them. This capacity for thought about feelings, which Bion called 'reverie', eventually creates the possibility for a withdrawal of the projections, allowing for mutual clarification of who is who in the interests of reality.

Summary

Counter-transference then, can be said to be an aspect of projective identification, indeed both Klein (1946, cited by Segal 1973) and Bion (1962) have identified it as being the result of projective identification. In counter-transference, the patient puts something into the therapist that the therapist experiences as his/her own. Projective identification splits off an unacceptable or undesirable (or uncontrollable) part of the self and puts it into another person. That person must have (if only to a very small degree) the potential to identify with, and express that feeling; it rises up from the general repertoire of that person's feelings and gets exaggerated and expressed. The projector can then feel: 'It's not me, it's him/her', while the process of identification in the recipient may yield a bewildering feeling, reaction or act. These projected emotions must find a suitable container to receive, identify and try to understand the emotions; something in the nurse that offers a home for the feelings being transferred from the patient.

An attempt has been made to interpret the literature surrounding the concepts of counter-transference and projective identification. The narrative described at the beginning of this chapter was initially difficult to relate in words and I made several attempts to capture the intensity of the atmosphere and emotions experienced by the participants at that particular time, but no words seemed capable of capturing the density and depth of the feelings. On re-reading, the narrative seems weak in its description. The ensuing attempt to interpret the content against the theory will hopefully enrich the description further.

Analysis

Analysis

The focus of the scenario is my relationship with John's mother. There were other relationships that affected me during this particular event. My working relationship with the doctor and his actions, which left me in a very difficult situation, caused me considerable anxiety and led me to question my professional integrity, but it is the relationship with John's mother that had the main impact on my functioning at this period. Never before, or since, have I experienced such an intense relationship with a carer of a patient. The relationship which was initially an easy going, relaxed, long-term relationship transformed very quickly into an uncomfortable, uncommunicative stand-off between myself and someone I thought I knew relatively well. It may have been the case that I identified with something in John, something about his history of self-harm and the potential gravity of the situation that was unfolding. To explore this however, would take me into my personal history which would be inappropriate here. Normally, I take the professional stance and feel that one must do one's best with patients, this time I felt extremely fearful and panicked and couldn't understand why I felt as I did. The focus of this discussion surrounds the events that got me in touch with the fragility of

Thoughts on the impact of a suicide

John's mother, as I attempted to recognise and compare the situation with the theories of counter-transference and projective identification.

My intuition was that John had died. I felt guilty that I felt that John had died. I felt guilty about the fact that I couldn't tell his mother that I thought he had died. I couldn't tell her this because I felt it would exacerbate the rapidly deteriorating relationship: that she would hate me for having this strong intuition, based on knowing John and probability. On reflection now, I feel that she knew I thought he would die, which is why she stayed on the ward and watched me, waiting for me to confirm her fears. I was failing to live up to the unshakeable belief that John's mother had in my ability to keep him safe and I was finding it uncomfortable and difficult to cope with or work through it. A question that springs to mind here is: Should we tell our patients about our intuitive thoughts and feelings? I feel that we shouldn't, if the thoughts/feelings are wrong, misjudgements might be made which could have damaging consequences for patients. The urge to speak to John's mother about my fears, about the possible scenario was, at times, almost overwhelming, but my fear of her reaction was more so. I wanted to tell her what I was thinking, that John was dead, that I feared he had taken his own life, but how do you say this to a parent, knowing that it may not be true? The parents had not even come to terms with John's diagnosis; how could they conceivably deal with his possible suicide? So I said nothing about my intuition.

I felt physically sick, and lost my appetite, I felt I had a weight in my stomach, a lead bar that stayed with me until sometime after John was found. I couldn't sleep or concentrate, my head and shoulders ached. I felt disillusioned with the system, the doctor had failed to take seriously my suspicion that John may attempt self-harm. I have a young son myself, the thought that I would see him grow up and destroy himself in such a way was underlying any discussions I had with John's mother. I was also quite fond of John, I had nursed him on more than one occasion and I was concerned for his safety.

John's mother visited every day until he was found, her presence on the ward seemed to perpetuate my feelings of hopelessness, guilt, sadness, and the feelings seemed more intense when she was there but were always present during those five days. My reactions appeared to particularly escalate just after I had spoken to John's mother. I can now identify these symptoms as being indications of an experience of projective identification.

John's mother was externally very calm while on the ward (I have no idea what she was like outside the ward environment); I felt her presence bore a silent reproach towards me and she continually stated that I would make everything right. She felt that I was able to make things better, I was the 'phantasy' figure that could make everything right. John's mother seemed to deny the reality of the situation, a position that might indicate fear, even terror of that reality. The panic, chaos and disintegration that I experienced were perhaps also projections from her. Maybe I was her container. Perhaps, she felt she was disintegrating and was only held together by the notion that I was to blame, not her. By bearing this, perhaps I did indeed help to hold it together for her. Her son seemed to be so central to her life, their life, as his parents.

Projective identification requires a splitting of the feelings experienced by the projector, a separation of the bad feelings from the good to protect the internal good object, thereby rescuing the individual from a feeling of self-destruction. So might splitting have occurred here? What were the bad feelings and where were they, what were the good feelings that were left in the mother? The bad feelings were the fear for John's safety, the responsibility for his situation, the panic and frustration at the lack of control and the feeling of futility. Perhaps John's mum was protecting herself by splitting her internal objects and ego into good and bad parts and projecting the bad parts into me. Initially it was a good part, containing all her hope that I would find her son, that he would be safe and I would restore him to her. Her love for John, combined with perhaps her hatred of him for being ill and leaving her, could have been separated so she would not be destroyed by the event. Perhaps she felt she was unable to accept John's illness because she was experiencing self-doubt and self-accusation that she had failed John in some way?

I question now why I allowed John's mother to remain on the ward during the five days prior to John being found. I wouldn't normally tolerate this. Something made me want her to be present. I felt then that I was empathising with her, that I knew how she was feeling and I felt sorry for her. It may have been the case that I was projecting into her, using her as a container for my own sense of guilt. I feel sympathy for any relative in this situation but it was this unshakeable belief in my ability and the strong physical and emotional feelings attached to this situation that made it different. I wonder now if I had turned her away, made her wait at home, if it would have made me feel better. I feel now that if I had, my reaction would probably have been similar but not as intense.

Giving meaning to the feelings

I can now give meaning to the feelings I experienced when with Mrs Smith. The potential loss of John must have been devastating, the parents' apparent denial of John's illness had, at last, been revealed and the truth realised. John was suffering from a mental illness which had possibly been the cause of his demise. The sense of failure and disappointment in John, and possibly in themselves as parents, combined with the fear, frustration and grief must have been immensely overwhelming. Mrs Smith seemed to have a figure that in her mind, or in her 'phantasy' could control the situation. I was always calm and confident in work, I knew my job and had a particularly good relationship with the family. I was fond of John, always looking out for him at meal and break times and interested in his general welfare. He and I often discussed music, we shared a liking for certain bands, my relationship with John could be said to have had maternal leanings.

I was probably the ideal recipient for Mrs Smith's projections. It could be said that we shared an identity in our roles of caring for John. This may have meant that we provided for each other a degree of mutual projection and identification. We had both looked after him when he was ill, both cared about his well-being; therefore, because of my relationship with John, I formed the ideal 'home' for her bad feelings, as indeed she may have done for some of mine.

At first I seemed idealised by the mother, with this feeling later turning to hate and my becoming an object of blame with the death of John. The initial idealisation of my abilities was reduced to denigration. Mrs Smith just walked away when I told her that John had been found, but the physical and emotional feelings I experienced remained with me for some time afterwards. I feel John's death was blamed on me because I was always the person who was able to make positive things happen and this time I failed to do this, I was not a perfect nurse or mother. I feel that had Mrs Smith reclaimed the feelings I was experiencing, I would then have been able to separate which feelings were hers and which were mine. If Mrs Smith had shouted at me or blamed me directly for what had happened, or even made a complaint about me, I think I would have felt it as just punishment. It would have absolved me of blame and the guilt I felt that I had failed. She would have been just another carer, the victim of tragic circumstance, venting her emotions on the nursing staff, staff who are paid and expected to take the brunt of emotional outpouring because that's what we do. But she just walked away. Spoken accusations are much easier to deal with than unspoken ones, the unspoken create a much greater sense of persecution and uncertainty.

I still feel the hate and blame emanating from the mother when I see her in the street, although there are no verbal exchanges of any type. This indicates that, if one accepts Bion's model of container/contained, I remain a container for her feelings.

Discussion

Discussion

By their very nature counter-transference and projective identification are unconscious processes, usually only discovered by reflection in the practitioner. Was it just that I felt vulnerable and genuinely afraid that I had been responsible for John's death? Was this the 'last straw' that broke down any ability to defend myself against my own feelings? In reality, and occasionally in the practice situation, the feelings that are provoked in everybody touched by suicide are similar to those I experienced in this situation: guilt, anger, sadness and pain. I thought at the time that I was just stressed by the situation. This form of stress and burn-out, in response to work pressures, can be a result of being the bearer of feelings and emotions, whose weight essentially belongs to the users of our service (Hughes and Pengelly, 1997).

As mentioned earlier in this chapter, some theorists (Ogden, 1979; Bateman and Holmes, 1995) claim that projective identification and counter-transference form part of a therapeutic relationship. Initially, this was difficult to find in relation to my scenario. The relationship didn't feel therapeutic, certainly from my perspective, but I now wonder what would have happened if the projection had not occurred. It may have led to John's mother becoming totally unable to cope and she might have become ill. I feel now that there was a projection of feelings for which I was a recipient, or a container. This revelation, or new understanding, now gives a degree of purpose to the whole incident, the event has become productive and, in a certain sense, even therapeutic for Mrs Smith and, from my perspective, has been therapeutic for me in helping to make sense of the event.

There is a possibility that because I am unfamiliar with the theory of projective identification and have never attempted to identify the process in interactions with patients previously, that I may have over-analysed this scenario. Initially, I thought that I was just empathising with Mrs Smith. Sutherland (1991) defines empathy as the capacity to participate in another's feelings and experiences and to understand them. The difference here is that I was actually experiencing the feelings that were being projected by Mrs Smith. The feelings were certainly experienced as being my own, I did not feel at any time that they could have come from anywhere else. In future practice, I would have to be aware of this possibility of misidentification.

Conclusion

This chapter has attempted to define and relate to practice the theories of counter-transference and projective identification. The examination of this scenario using these theories has helped to translate the 'way I felt' into 'why I felt as I did'. This event occurred just over three years ago, looking at the event in the light of reading key theorists has deepened my understanding of the incident and my reaction. Smith and Nursten (1995, cited by Hughes and Pengelly 1997) suggest that practitioners may need repeated opportunities over a number of years to reflect on the impact of an event, as the capacity for understanding deepens with increasing distance from the incident.

The application of the theories explored here has helped with my interpretation of the impact of this event and the whole scenario has been transformed into a purposeful incident which makes the physical and emotional experience easier to bear.

Putting the incident into words, describing emotions and attempting to apply meaning to them has helped make sense of what and why this happened.

Some might feel that a suicide is a difficult enough issue to be exposed to at the best of times; suicide is not common in the field of mental health nursing, although one could say one suicide is too many, but still it is an issue that mental health nurses face every working day. With this in mind, suicide still has a considerable impact on everyone involved. That someone would want to take their own life, regardless of the impact of this act on everyone who cares for them, results in shock, anger, frustration and confusion. These emotions added to the turmoil of this particular situation. Despite all my best efforts at being a nurse, and a surrogate carer for John, the system (and I) failed to keep him safe. The blame and guilt attached to this failure complicated my freedom to think about John's mother's experience as a separate experience. This slight confusion made me a good recipient for her projections, and also made it hard for me to sort out what was 'me' and what was 'her'. I now feel this confusion has, to some extent, been explained.

References

Bateman, A. and Holmes, J. (1995). *Introduction to Psychoanalysis: Contemporary Theory and Practice*. London: Routledge.

Bion, R.W. (1962). *Learning from Experience*. London: Heinemann.

Hinshelwood, R.D. (1991). *A Dictionary of Kleinian Thought*, 2nd edn. London: Free Association Books.

Hughes, L. and Pengelly, P. (1997). *Staff Supervision in a Turbulent Environment*. London: Jessica Kingsley.

Ogden, T.K. (1979). 'On projective identification.' *International Journal of Psychoanalysis* 60: 357–3.

O'Kelly, G. (1998). 'Countertransference in the nurse-patient relationship: a review of the literature.' *Journal of Advanced Nursing* 28(2): 391–7.

Schroder, P.J. (1985). 'Recognising transference and countertransference.' *Journal of Psychosocial Nursing* 23(2): 21–6.

Segal, H. (1973). *Introduction to the Work of Melanie Klein*. London: Hogarth.

Sutherland, S. (1991). *Dictionary of Psychology*. London: MacMillan.

Winnicott, D.W. (1947). 'Hate in the countertransference.' *International Journal of Psychoanalysis* 30: 69–74.

Commentary on 'Joe's story' & 'The impact of a suicide'

**Commentary on 'Joe's story'
and 'The impact of a suicide'**
Louise de Raeve

I have chosen to comment on these chapters together because I was struck by their similarities as well as differences. Despite the fact that Mary writes about a patient dying on a general ward and Alyson about a suicide in a psychiatric hospital, both chapters take the nurse to the edge of her capacity to manage, both involve a death and both are primarily about the reaction of a key relative. Both also explore projective identification, with Alyson's chapter linking this explicitly with the idea of counter-transference and Mary's chapter leaving this as implicit. These are not everyday nursing experiences: the relatives' reactions and the nurses' emotional responses to them are very hard for these experienced nurses to bear, in some ways even impossible. The words used bear testimony to this. Alyson writes: 'The sense of panic, fear, hopelessness and frustration stayed with me over the next few days and I was having difficulty sleeping, doing, thinking about anything other than John and his probable fate'. Mary writes: 'Earlier … I stated that I felt affronted by Mrs D's accusations that I was trying to kill Joe … In retrospect, I think better words would be panicky, bewildered, misunderstood and scared'.

'Frozen grief' is a phrase that comes to mind thinking about these chapters. Each death is a terrible threat: untimely, unimaginable from Mrs D's perspective and from Mrs Smith's, shocking and sudden. Neither relative seems to have been able to take in the severity of the illness their loved-one suffered from, leaving them completely unprepared for this possible consequence. The chapter writers draw our attention to this denial and to the difficulties of helping someone in this state of mind. Everyone seems locked into a persecutory frame of thinking, where blame and guilt predominate, real communication falters and nurses are watching their backs for fear of accusations: murder in Mary's case, negligence in Alyson's. There is no ceiling to these ideas, they spiral in a confusion of fantasy and reality. The hospital experience seems to persecute these relatives and in their turn they persecute the nurse with overt or silent accusations. This is the world of the paranoid-schizoid position, as described by Melanie Klein (1988) where splitting and projection abound and real mourning cannot happen. Alyson and Mary would have had no choice in being caught up in this.

These are very powerful processes and it would take more than a single individual to 'hold' or contain this experience. Sadly, institutional wisdom, which might have supported these nurses better, seems to have left them standing rather alone. There was some response, but for Alyson, the 'sticking plaster' gesture failed to grasp what she felt she was up against and for Mary, the response may have unwittingly confirmed Mrs D's view of events and left Joe dying in distress.

Mary's and Alyson's narratives are, I believe, attempts to try and digest what happened, to see meaning in what could at the time only be survived. This is to try to move towards the depressive position. This journey is particularly difficult in a situation which cannot be repaired in actuality but only internally, by an internal adjustment. These nurses, I think, have had to bear being a 'bad object' for these relatives, without redemption and it is interesting that Alyson wonders if this in itself may have been helpful for John's mother, helping her hold herself together. We cannot know if this was so but it may well be true. Both Alyson and Mary were unconsciously required to contain enormous rage and hatred. They did, to the best of their respective abilities, and sometimes surviving in the face of such challenges is all one can do. I believe it must be excruciatingly difficult for Alyson to have to encounter Mrs Smith in her daily life, a constant reminder of this state of affairs, and maybe it is equally hard for Mrs Smith. The only way one can deal with this sort of situation is not to take it personally. Whoever Alyson is for Mrs Smith, it is not Alyson herself that is being related to in this way but beyond this we cannot know. Mary writes about the tendency to avoid the discomfort that contact with Mrs D produced, by having as little to do with her as was necessary. Without other resources to help understand what was happening, this is what occurs, nurses withdraw, but it can mean that the most needy patients and relatives get less care than they warrant and it could be interpreted by such patients/relatives as punishment; sometimes this may even be the intention. In this way persecutory situations escalate.

Commentary on 'Joe's story' & 'The impact of a suicide'

With the wisdom of hindsight, it is easy to say that both these relatives show signs of great vulnerability: they would rank highly in a bereavement risk assessment, as being in need of professional support, which of course they might have refused if it had been offered, and maybe it was, we have no way of knowing.

It takes courage to write about and publish a nursing encounter that felt far from ideal and also where there are no neat solutions to tidy everything up. The theoretical perspective may help bear it but it does not remove the anguish. What one can see though, vividly described, is how difficult nursing is, that it can push good nurses to the limits of their professional and personal capacities. If we want people to keep thinking and not to withdraw in such very difficult circumstances, we need to provide the institutional structures that can truly assist nurses to hold on to their professional selves in an emotionally alive way, thereby enabling them to deliver the best care they are capable of.

The third and final section in the book responds to this issue. It contains three chapters; the first gives an overview of the research literature that supports the utility of a psychodynamic way of thinking. The second chapter is a summary of a research project that assessed the effectiveness of group supervision for a group of palliative care nurses. Psychodynamic thinking was the main, explanatory theory chosen to assist with understanding what took place in the small group and the research analysis that was conducted subsequently. The last chapter offers a psychodynamic framework for clinical supervision, using Winnicott's (1990) concepts of handling, holding and object presenting.

References

Klein, M. (1988). *Envy and Gratitude and Other Works 1946–1963*. London: Virago (chapters 1 and 6 in particular).

Winnicott, D.W. (1990). 'Ego integration in child development' [1962]. In *The Maturational Processes and the Facilitating Environment*. London: Karnac, pp.56–63.

Part III

The wider context
Research and supervision

Chapter 12
Reviewing the evidence base for psychodynamic principles in nursing
Heather Davies

Introduction

It has long been recognised that evidence-based practice within health care is important to ensure that patients benefit to the greatest extent possible from the treatments they receive and, particularly, do not come to any harm as a result of their care. Strauss *et al.* (2004) state that evidence-based health care is the integration of individual clinical expertise with the best available external clinical evidence from systematic research, including patients' values and expectations. The evidence base in health care is variable, with evidence of treatments that are helpful as well as those that are harmful to patients. However, for the most part in health care, it is not known whether the care given is of benefit, only that it appears to do no harm. Consequently, the current aim of evidence-based practice is to increase the knowledge base, thereby eliminating harmful treatments and determining the effects of other treatments. In this way, it is hoped that the clinical effectiveness of care will be maximised.

It is particularly difficult to demonstrate the effects of interactions between the healthcare professional and the individual receiving care. Healthcare literature is littered with advice on the need for good communication and psychological care, but evidence-based examples of how this is best achieved are scant. This chapter will consider issues surrounding the provision of an evidence base for psychological care in nursing, with particular emphasis on the evidence for using a psychodynamic approach.

Nurses and their patients

Evidence-based practice

There are a number of considerations in evaluating the evidence in relation to health care. One is the distinction between efficacy and effectiveness (Cochrane, 1972). Efficacy determines whether a specific treatment works and often refers to evidence derived from carefully designed trials, where threat to internal validity is minimised. Effectiveness relates to whether treatments that have been tested work in everyday practice. Evidence may be in the form of a report of validated research, often distilled into clinical guidelines, for consideration in relation to personal and best practice. In the past, clinical guidelines have been developed by professional bodies or selected experts in the field but the introduction of the National Institute for Clinical Excellence (NICE) ensures that there is a mechanism by which guidelines can be approved, disseminated and adopted throughout the National Health Service (Department of Health, 2008).

A dilemma when considering evidence-based practice is what constitutes evidence. While it is generally accepted that the types of available evidence will differ according to the sort of treatment being evaluated, there is also a generally accepted hierarchy for assessing evidence as shown in Table 12.1.

Table 12.1　　**Hierarchy for assessing evidence**

LEVEL 1	Randomised controlled trials
↓	Cohort studies
	Case control studies
	Consensus statements
LEVEL 5	Expert opinion

The hierarchy guides the judgement of best evidence. Level 1 evidence is thought to be the randomised controlled trial, where the impact of treatment is determined by randomly allocating two matched groups of people to receive different therapies and evaluating the effects of treatment. The randomised controlled trial is considered to be the 'gold standard' because of its ability to deal with bias through the randomisation process. However, even with the randomised controlled trial, there may be a trade-off between rigour and generalisability (Shapiro *et al.*, 1994; 1995). The more selective the sample and rigorously defined the intervention, the more applicable the research may be to particular patients and the less applicable the treatment may be in practice.

Other levels of evidence are as described, down to Level 5, which is based on expert opinion or consensus in the absence of formal critical appraisal (NHS Centre for Reviews and Dissemination, 1999). In effectiveness research, the design is weighted towards high generalisability, but a price is paid in terms of internal validity and being able to demonstrate that treatment has caused the changes claimed. New treatments can be tested for efficacy, and then introduced and tested for effectiveness in practice to ensure evidence-based practice (Barkham and Mellor-Clark, 2000). However, the length of time, from the development of a new treatment to its adoption into routine practice, means that treatments are often being modified in the light of new research by the time they are in general use (Margison *et al.*, 1998).

So it is clear that while evidence-based practice may be the aim of modern health care, it is often hard to demonstrate. If this is so with treatments that lend themselves relatively easily to scientific research methods, how much more difficult will it be for those where effects are likely to be due to many factors in care. Application of evidence-based practice to the nurse–patient relationship, including psychological interventions, is complex. The evidence base for psychotherapy has been extensively reviewed and is weighted towards those treatments that lend themselves to quantitative data collection, such as cognitive behavioural therapy. A lack of evidence concerning many therapies is revealed, rather than evidence for or against (Roth and Fonagy, 1996).

Margison *et al.* (1998) argue that the problem with measuring psychotherapeutic interventions using randomised controlled trials is the difficulty in applying them to individual cases. This often results in the conclusion that any intervention is better than none, rather than assessment of the value of a particular therapy. Richardson (2001) undertook a cogent review of the difficulties associated with assessing the effectiveness of psychodynamic therapy, highlighting problems in deciding the outcome measures to be assessed, the long-term nature of psychological therapies and the individuality of both client and patient, as confounding variables. He concluded that despite this, ongoing studies are being conducted and in future, more evidence may be available.

When considering measurement of effectiveness within the nurse–patient relationship, through the accepted hierarchy of evidence, more problems arise. It is generally accepted that nursing practice needs to be informed by research evidence, what is widely questioned, however, is what constitutes 'evidence'. An exploration of some of the issues may shed more light on what may be important to consider and what evidence is available.

The development of nursing knowledge

Nursing knowledge

One dilemma when assessing the evidence for nursing interventions is that much credence is currently given to the work of both Carper (1978) on ways of knowing and Benner and Wrubel (1989) on intuitive knowledge. Benner and Wrubel (1982) describe clinical knowledge as that embedded in the practice of nursing. They discuss the differences between 'knowing that' (theoretical knowledge) and 'knowing how' (practical knowledge) as explicated by the philosophers of science Polanyi (1962) and Kuhn (1962). Skilled practice may be based on tacit knowledge, that is, it may not involve explicit knowledge of the underlying theoretical principles. It is therefore difficult to assess by objective measurement (Polanyi, 1962). Polanyi (1962) describes those who use such implicit skills as connoisseurs, where qualitative, critical, discriminative judgements are made. Skilled knowledge allows the nurse a perceptual grasp of the situation because of previous experience. It relies on perceptual awareness that distinguishes relevant from irrelevant information and grasps the whole situation, rather than a series of tasks. This is accomplished rapidly, without deliberate analysis of individual factors and is developed through experience. Knowledge about individual parts of the situation is not necessary to understand it, although may be needed to determine a solution. This level of skill is described by Benner and Wrubel (1982) as expert practice, where theory is refined through practice and past experience used as paradigm cases. Benner and Wrubel (1989) assert that excellence is embodied in practice and is a moral art, not an applied science. However, this type of knowledge is often not established or tested through quantitative methodology.

Argyris and Schön (1974) developed the idea of 'theory in use' where practitioners share their actions in relation to a practice situation and seek to identify the theories used, generated by their experience, education, values and beliefs. These theories are often implicit in spontaneous behaviour and only apparent on reflection, or when a person has to think deliberately about what to do in relation to a particular problem encountered. Practice is advocated as a basis for learning and understanding care. This may be particularly important when considering evidence of patient experience and improvement in the patient's psychological state and may provide the evidence base for aspects of care that involve interaction between a healthcare professional and patient. Further, many, if not all, aspects of the nurse–patient relationship can only be researched using a qualitative research approach, as outcomes are attributable to a number of factors other than the patient's relationship with the nurse.

There are further difficulties in applying a quantitative approach to researching the nurse–patient relationship. These, notably, are the ethical difficulties created by the development of a relationship that is not chosen but comes about through a need for care, leading to a lack of patient consent to different psychological approaches. Shortage of time in acute settings makes randomisation and quantitative research challenging to set up and also there are problems in reducing the variables when at least two people are involved and bring their own personalities and motivations to the relationship. Nursing is primarily interested in the whole experience of the patient, rather than cause and effect or intervention results as in medicine. Understanding a patient's experience of illness provides insight into how to care for other patients in similar circumstances, so nursing research needs to focus on the reality of each patient's situation. Therefore, evidence relevant to nursing needs to be generated, using research, but also by other techniques, for example, reflection and considering case studies.

Nurses and their patients

Nursing practice and the nurse–patient relationship have developed, largely through practitioners sharing their practice and patients telling their stories. Jones (1995) describes a case study illustrating the use of Peplau's (1988) model in caring for a man who had had a cerebral vascular accident, providing an interesting example of case study research. The single case study method informs practice by illustrating dilemmas and issues in practice and helps in the development of alternative therapeutic responses. Psychodynamic approaches (Malan, 1995, Storr, 2002), person-centred approaches (Rogers, 1951), Gestalt, cognitive behavioural (Grant *et al.*, 2004) have all used single case studies as evidence for theory. However, case studies are often questioned as a method because they are incapable of providing generalisable conclusions (Tellis, 1997). The single case could be considered acceptable, provided it met recognised processes of assessment of rigour in qualitative methodology and it was accepted that outcomes from individual case studies are analytically generalisable but not statistically generalisable (Polit *et al.*, 2006).

Currently, there is little gold standard evidence for assessing the effectiveness of the relationship and interactions between nurse and patient and, as discussed, there are difficulties in using a quantitative research approach to improve the situation. However, gathering good-quality data from routine practice, leading to practice-based evidence may overcome some of the problems, although in the hierarchy of evidence this type of research is not highly rated. Both the value of psychodynamic therapies and nurse–patient relationships are, for the most part, poorly empirically supported, using the accepted criteria (Table 12.1) for contemporary reviews. There is some merit for the use of qualitative research studies, as a basis for evidence-based practice in nursing.

The nurse–patient relationship

Nurse–patient relationship

The interpersonal relationship between nurse and patient often provides the energy, motivation and source of strength for the patient to undergo their suffering (Chambers, 2006) and is crucial if the meaning of patients' individual suffering is to be identified, and relief provided. The nurse–patient relationship is often heightened during physical or psychological crisis, when the patient is especially vulnerable. Therapeutic relationships are considered important for those experiencing threats to their health and aim to initiate supportive interpersonal communication, so as to understand the perceptions and needs of the other person, empowering them to cope more effectively with their environment and resolve problems (Forchuk and Reynolds, 2001). They differ from social relationships in terms of goals, in that the nurse–patient relationship may have mutually agreed aims but social relationships are more spontaneous. While both involve personal disclosure and intimacy, only a therapeutic relationship has the aim of facilitating recovery or adjustment from illness (Peplau, 1988). In considering the existing evidence relating to the nurse–patient relationship, there seem to be three main areas of interest: the approach taken to the nurse–patient relationship, nurse motivation and difficulties, and the way that nurses cope with these.

Development of the nurse–patient relationship is known to be a complicated process that places demands on the nurse to have excellent communication skills and to become involved with patients in their care (Skilbeck and Payne, 2003). The nurse must gain information about the patient to determine care needs. Peplau (1988) emphasises intuitive or non-verbal communication in this process of coming to know the person. She places stress on lasting involvement, based on skills of empathy, judgement and the ability to see what is needed. Meutzel (1988) also discusses the nurse–patient relationship as a therapeutic process, highlighting intimacy, partnership and reciprocity as key concepts. Both Meutzel (1988) and Peplau (1988) emphasise the importance of encouraging the patient to find their own solutions to problems, through a non-directive approach to care and the nurse–patient relationship. The aims are clear but it can be challenging for nurses to achieve a therapeutic nurse–patient relationship with every patient (Heaven and Maguire, 1996; Moyle, 2003). There are motivations and tensions on both sides and self-awareness is crucial for managing the relationship and the level of involvement. This is especially true when the nurse is dealing with patients who are very emotionally or physically distressed.

There seems to be little research within the nursing literature, testing approaches taken towards psychological care and the nurse–patient relationship but there is some that provides insight into the factors and processes involved. Ramos (1992), Morse (1991) and May (1991) undertook detailed qualitative studies of the nurse–patient relationship and showed that the most beneficial nurse–patient relationships are those that are patient-, rather than nurse-led. Reciprocity and attachment affect the nurse–patient relationship positively when present, increasing benefits to both parties, but reciprocity and involvement are also problematic. It is evident that, while nurses may gain from the nurse–patient relationship, reward is not to be expected and there is a fine line between a productive nurse–patient relationship that allows intimacy and involvement on the part of both nurse and patient, and one that is not functioning.

Mok and Chiu (2004) found that the nurse–patient relationship in palliative care consisted of four main processes of *encountering in the caring process, forming a trusting and connected relationship, refilling fuel and being enriched*. Trust, caring and reciprocity were important elements of the nurse–patient relationship and there was involvement of both nurse and patient. Care and sharing meant that both patients and nurses found meaning in palliative care, which involves sharing the suffering of patients and the continual development of relationships that will be broken with the patient's death. Many nurses describe intense emotions in response to their clinical encounters (Cohen, 1995). De Araujo and da Silva (2004) in a small qualitative study to discover how nurses cope with daily confrontation with death and dying patients, found that dealing with the suffering of patients and their families produced feelings of depression and melancholy in the nurses and that they felt the suffering of their patients. Rowe (2003) identifies reverberations with the past, expectations, guilt, vulnerability, the high cost of empathy, inflicting pain, silence and the healer's spiritual or philosophical beliefs, as sources of threat to those who are caring for suffering people.

Paley *et al.* (2003) implemented training for a small group of mental health nurses in the Hobson (1985) Conversational Model of therapy (also known as psychodynamic-interpersonal therapy), an integrative model of therapy that combines psychodynamic, humanistic, and interpersonal theory and techniques, based on developing a relationship between therapist and client around negotiation. The model has been extensively researched and shown to be effective for mental health and physical problems (Shapiro *et al.*, 1994, Guthrie *et al.*, 1998, Meares *et al.*, 1999). Paley *et al.* (2003) found that the nurses were able to use the approach successfully, although organisational pressures caused some difficulties.

There are some studies that indicate that the attachment style of patients affects their response to care (see Chapter 2). Attachment security can act as a buffer to depressive symptoms in patients with metastatic cancer (Rodin *et al.*, 2007, Brennan *et al.*, 1998). Griffin and Bartholomew (1994) found that dismissing attachment style was associated with worse compliance to medical regimens and could be mediated by the patient–provider relationship. Ciechanowski *et al.* (2004) found a significant degree of variance in adherence to recommended medication for diabetes that may be mediated by attachment style. When empathy and responsiveness were shown by clinicians, patients' participation and autonomy in decision making increased. The positive influence of a collaborative, patient–provider relationship also improved compliance to prescribed treatment. Feeney (2000) argued that measurement of attachment security in children affects responses to pain, illness, emotional regulation and utilisation of resources. She stressed the importance for health professionals to consider attachment as a multidimensional construct that affects emotional regulation and how individuals respond fundamentally to caregivers. Awareness of this enables interactions to be adjusted according to patients' levels of dependence and anxiety. However, she acknowledged the methodological difficulties of measuring attachment in sick children, as parents' responses can influence results. This could also be said of adults undergoing personal trauma which changes their existing close relationships. Odegard (2005) worked with potential disruptions to attachment imposed by chronic illness in children and noted three critical elements in the attachment process to address this; *holding, containing*, and *the provision of space*. She acknowledged that clinicians can have a tendency to take control, because of their own anxiety. This can block the provision of space, impair parental confidence and lead to greater dependency.

The complexities involved in the nurse–patient relationship mean that self-awareness and awareness of patient reactions is crucial. The nurse must be able to practice without becoming overwhelmed by either her own or the patient's emotions. There are many motivations for nurses' responses to the patient's plight. Empathy is considered important to ensure a connection to the patient; sympathy and empathy may motivate one to help another but empathy enables the response to be patient-led and is about patients' feelings rather than nurses' (Rogers, 1951). Sympathy is the carer's response to another's plight (Morse, 2006) and can be seen as *having pity for*. In sympathy a personal emotional response is evoked that is not detached and is about the individual's feelings in response to another's distress. Sympathy may motivate others to care (Wispe, 1986, Travelbee, 1972) or interfere with their ability to help (Forsyth, 1979).

The ability to respond to another may depend on the extent to which one infers another's affective state and self-awareness is important for patient-focused empathy, with reflection needed, to evaluate what the experience means for nurse and patient (Thompson, 1996). However, Morse *et al.* (1992, 2006) argue that it is not always possible to have an empathic relationship with the patient and that at times, sympathy is more appropriate. Empathy in clinical practice was explored and it was found that learned therapeutic empathy, as advocated in counselling, where the aim is to help the person gain insight, is not appropriate when working with patients who are suffering. Emotive engagement or the intuitive sensing and response to another's plight is more apt, and patients often need sympathy and pity. Morse *et al.* (1992, 2006) maintained that emotional empathy is learned through experience and modelling, and that nurses know implicitly what to do when a patient is distressed.

There are difficulties when nurses over-identify with the patient and are arguably motivated by sympathy rather than empathy. Davies (2007) undertook a phenomenological study of thirty-one experienced palliative care clinical nurse specialists, to determine their understanding and management of patient suffering. She found a high level of self-awareness among the nurses who knew that, at times, and with different patients, their response was empathic and, at others, sympathetic. They also knew that they would have a more intimate relationship with some patients and were aware that, if they could identify with a patient, it would affect their care. In some situations, the palliative care nurse specialists did not seem to be making a judgement based on the patient's needs, but on their own imagined responses, as if they were going through the same experience. Omdahl and O'Donnell (1999) propose that to reduce nursing burnout, education needs to help nurses effectively communicate, differentiate between empathic concern and emotional contagion and identify when they are experiencing each. Effective strategies should be promoted to enhance empathic concern and reduce emotional contagion (Omdahl and O'Donnell, 1999).

Prolonged stress resulting from caring can lead to complete emotional blocking on the part of the caregiver, who becomes completely detached from the sufferer. Morse *et al.* (2006) describe the ways in which distance is created by shielding, withdrawing and guarding which reduce the caregiver's sensitivity to the sufferer's experience. This may lead to labelling, dehumanising, distancing and denying, which change the caregiver's perception of suffering. The resulting detachment enables the caregiver to continue to give care and manage the resulting stress. However, the caregiver's responses are repressed and a front is presented to the patient, who may be aware that they are not being treated as an individual.

Therapeutic nurse–patient relationships depend on the ability of the nurse to comprehend the subjective world of the patient (Chapter 5 gives an illustration of this). Nurses try to protect themselves from being overwhelmed with emotions, by distancing themselves from the situation and by focusing on tasks to be performed or sharing the care burden with colleagues. Georges *et al.* (2002) found that nurses working in palliative care tried to remain authentic and stay close to patients, even when they could not alleviate their problems, although this approach was less commonly adopted than one of 'distancing'. The nurses recognised the pain of caring for patients who are dying and tried to preserve themselves, while also trying to help the patient. Rittman *et al.* (1997) discussed how nurses limit their relationships with patients to protect themselves from excessive emotional demands, an argument supported by the work of Payne *et al.* (1998) who found that nurses focused on physical care, thus protecting themselves from patients' emotional reactions.

Studies have shown that patient communication skills, expression of appreciation for nursing care, ability to get on with others and similarity in values, all affect the nurse–patient relationship (Jarrett and Payne, 1995, Johnson and Webb, 1995, Kahn and Steeves, 1988, Forrest, 1989). Further, the patient's ability to take responsibility for their illness or change their behaviour affects the way nurses respond to them (Morrison, 1990, Olsen, 1997). Where patients are unable to do so constructively, due to dementia or other illness, this can result in their nurses being less tolerant of them (Morrison, 1990, Olsen, 1997). Patients who do not take advice and fail to improve are considered hard to care for, which can lead to distancing or burn out (Finlay, 1997). Menzies' (1970) seminal work on responding to patients has been repeated and it is clear that nurses distance themselves from patients that they find difficult (Morse, 2006, Turner, 2001, Davies, 2007).

However, over-involvement can result in the nurses' excessive need to control and dominate the situation to protect their own interests, and this hinders patient recovery. Boundaries between self and others are blurred, and the carer may become an omnipotent rescuer, rather than allowing the person to take responsibility and use their own resources. Symptoms of counter-transference are over-involvement (Hartman, 1995), withdrawal from a patient (Holden, 1990) and the 'just a routine' approach to patient care (Yuen, 1986). O'Kelly (1998), reviewing the literature on counter-transference in nursing, promotes the importance of recognising counter-transference. She claims such recognition results in professional and personal growth in the nurse and advocates clinical supervision as a way to help nurses achieve this (endorsed by many chapters in this book).

The more experience and knowledge a nurse has, the better able they seem to be at managing their involvement. As they develop maturity, they become more aware of the effects of their behaviour, both on themselves and those around them (Turner, 2001, Davies, 2007). Nurses' ability to distance themselves from their patients develops over time and is necessary to protect them from being emotionally overwhelmed (Rittman *et al.*, 1997, Rasmussen *et al.* 1997, Payne *et al.*, 1998, Payne 2001). Turner (2001), in a grounded research study of oncology nurses, developed a theory of managing involvement. She identified 'becoming involved', 'experiencing over-involvement', 'developing awareness', 'controlling involvement' and 'being involved'. Two particular strategies were employed: the first, *setting boundaries*, enabled nurses to make a conscious decision about how far they would take their personal involvement. The second, *switching off*, meant that nurses stopped thinking about work when they went home and were able to get on with life outside. Graham (2005) undertook a study to uncover the meaning of the 'lived experience' of mutual suffering in relation to the care of a dying patient. He found that mutual suffering is a transformational process, leading to professional confusion and personal crisis, but that it involves new beginnings and clarification of beliefs and values.

The case for clinical supervision

The case for clinical supervision

It is clear that the dynamic between nurse and patient is a critical factor in the relationship, resulting in both effectiveness and difficulty for the nurse. Self- and patient-awareness are crucial and clinical supervision may be a way of learning from practice and developing the skills necessary for managing the relationship. Developing this may only be possible, using knowledge from practice and reflection on, and in, practice. Clinical supervision may provide the vehicle for this reflection, thereby assisting learning, as well as coping with difficult clinical situations.

The potential benefits of good clinical supervision undertaken by experienced supervisors and the use of psychodynamic principles to underpin the process are discussed by de Raeve (1998). She describes practice examples where nurses have been in difficult situations with patients who are angry or afraid and their reported emotions and reactions when dealing with these circumstances. An understanding of the motivations for patient reactions may help nurses to come to terms with events but also to learn for the future. This does of course require experience and knowledge of psychological dynamics on the part of the supervisor, who may also be learning through their work. Jones (2003) undertook a research study of five nurses working in palliative care, using qualitative methodology to determine the effects of small group work discussion. He explained his findings, using a psychoanalytic approach and an account of this research is to be found in the next chapter.

Rafferty (2000) discussed Winnicott's (1960) concepts of 'holding', 'handling' and 'object presenting', as a framework for clinical supervision, with the supervisor providing the 'mothering' required for growth of the nurse caring for patients. He presented the problems currently associated with clinical supervision in practice and argued that a supervisor, working within a theoretical framework outlined by Winnicott (1960), could be helpful. A version of this paper forms the last chapter in this book. Rafferty and de Raeve's (1998) work are examples of where evidence is largely derived from practice rather than quantitative research.

Conclusion

This chapter has explored some evidence supporting the use of a psychodynamic approach to understand nurse–patient relationships and interactions. Such an approach requires considerable self-knowledge and theoretical understanding on the part of the nurse and the development of these could be assisted through clinical supervision. There is some limited research relating to the nurse–patient relationship currently available, however using quantitative methodology to provide evidence is challenging for this type of care. The 'quantitative versus qualitative' debate is somewhat sterile and using whatever approaches are relevant to the clinical problem may be more appropriate for considering psychological interventions. Evidence from clinical practice can be subjected to critical review, both for verification at the individual level and potential transferability to other settings. Although this does not conform to traditional notions of reliability and validity, it may conform to rigour within the qualitative method. Ryecroft-Malone et al. (2004) suggested that robustness of professional knowledge, via reflection on case studies, can be established by gathering evidence from clinical practice and determining its impact on patients, colleagues and the organisation. The challenge is to ensure that methodological approaches are as rigorous as possible, whilst also ensuring that individualised care is delivered.

References

Argyris, C. and Schon, D. (1974). *Theory in Practice: Increasing Professional Effectiveness*. Massachusetts: Addison-Wesley.

Barkham, M. and Mellor-Clark, J. (2000). 'Rigour and relevance: practice-based evidence in the psychological therapies.' In *Evidence-based Health Care in Psychological Therapies*. Eds. N. Rowland and S. Goss. London: Routledge, pp.127–44.

Benner, P. and Wrubel, J. (1982). 'Skilled clinical knowledge: the value of perpetual awareness'. *Nurse Educator,* May–June: 11–17

Benner, P. and Wrubel, J. eds. (1989). *The Primacy of Caring: Stress and Coping in Health and Illness*. Menlo Park, CA: Addison Wesley.

Brennan, K.A., Clark, C.L. and Shaver, P.R. (1998). 'Self report measurement of adult romantic attachment: an integrative overview.' In *Attachment Theory and Close Relationships*, eds. J.A. Simpson and W.S. Rholes. New York: Guilford Press.

Carper, B. (1978). 'Fundamental patterns of knowing.' *Advances in Nursing Science* 1: 13–23.

Chambers, M. (2006). 'A concept analysis of therapeutic relationships.' In *The Essential Concepts of Nursing*, eds. J. Cutliffe and H.P. McKenna. Edinburgh: Elsevier, Churchill-Livingstone.

Ciechanowski, P., Russo, J., Katon, W., Von Korff, M., Ludman, E., Lin, E., Simon, G. and Bush, T. (2004). 'Influence of patient attachment style on self-care and outcomes in diabetes.' *Psychosomatic Medicine* 66: 720–8.

Cochrane, A.L. (1972). *Effectiveness and Efficiency. Random Reflections on Health Services*. London: Nuffield Provincial Hospitals Trust.

Cohen, M.Z. (1995). 'The meaning of cancer and oncology nursing: link to effective care.' *Seminars in Oncology Nursing* 11(1): 59–67.

Davies, H.M. (2007). 'Palliative care nurse specialists' understanding and management of suffering and their individual response to working with patients who are suffering: an investigation.' Unpublished D.Nurs.Sci. study: University of Wales, Swansea.

De Araujo, M.M.T. and da Silva, M.J.P. (2004). 'Nursing the dying: essential elements in the care of terminally ill patients.' *International Nursing Review* 51(3): 149–58.

De Raeve, L. (1998). 'Maintaining integrity through clinical supervision.' *Nursing Ethics* 5: 486–96.

Department of Health (2008). *High Quality Care for All: NHS next stage final review report*. London: Department of Health.

Feeney, J.A. (2000). 'Implications of attachment style for patterns of health and illness.' *Child: Care, Health and Development* 26 (4): 277–88.

Finlay, L. (1997). 'Good patients and bad patients: how occupational therapists view their patients and clients.' *British Journal of Occupational Therapy* 60: 440–6.

Forchuk, C. and Reynolds, W. (2001). 'Guest editorial – interpersonal theory in nursing practice, the Peplau legacy.' *Journal of Psychiatric and Mental Health Nursing* 5: 165–6.

Forrest, D. (1989). 'The experience of caring.' *Journal of Advanced Nursing* 14: 815–23.

Forsyth, G.L. (1979). 'Exploration of empathy in nurse-client interaction.' *Advances in Nursing Science* 1(2): 53–61.

Georges, J., Grypdonc, M. and De Casterle, B.D. (2002). 'Being a palliative care nurse in an academic hospital: a qualitative study about nurses' perceptions of palliative care nursing.' *Journal of Clinical Nursing* 11: 785–93.

Graham, I.W. (2005). 'Mutual suffering: a nurse's story of caring for the living as they are dying.' *International Journal of Nursing Practice* 11(6): 277–85.

Grant, A., Mills, J., Mulhern, R. and Short, M. (2004). *Cognitive Behavioural Therapy in Mental Health Care*. London: Sage Publications.

Griffin, D.W. and Bartholomew, K. (1994). 'The metaphysics of measurement: the case of adult attachment.' *Advances in Personal Relationships* 5: 17–52.

Guthrie, E., Moorey, J., Barker, H., Margison, F. and McGrath, G. (1998). 'Brief psychodynamic-interpersonal therapy for patients with severe psychiatric illness which is unresponsive to treatment.' *British Journal of Psychotherapy* 15: 155–66.

Hartman, C.R. (1995). 'The nurse patient relationship and victims of violence.' *Scholarly Inquiry for Nursing Practice*, 175–92.

Heaven, C.M. and Maguire, P. (1996). 'Training hospice nurses to elicit patient concerns.' *Journal of Advanced Nursing* 23: 280–6.

Hobson, R.F. (1985). *Forms of Feeling: The Heart of Psychotherapy*. London: Routledge.

Holden, R.J. (1990). 'Models, muddles and medicine.' *International Journal for Nursing Studies* 27(3): 223–34.

Jarrett, N. and Payne, S. (1995). 'A selective review of the literature on nurse–patient communication: has the patient's contribution been neglected?' *Journal of Advanced Nursing* 22: 72–8.

Johnson, M. and Webb, C. (1995). 'Rediscovering unpopular patients: the concept of social judgment.' *Journal of Advanced Nursing* 21(3): 466–75.

Jones, A. (1995). 'Utilizing Peplau's psychodynamic theory for stroke patient care'. *Journal of Clinical Nursing* 4(1): 49–54.

Jones, A. (2003). 'On projective identification, containment, and feeling special: Some thoughts about hospice nurses' experiences.' *American Journal of Hospice Palliative Care* 20(6): 441–46.

Kahn, D. and Steeves, R. (1988). 'Caring and practice: construction of the nurses' world.' *Scholarly Inquiry for Nursing Practice* 2: 201–21.

Kuhn, T.S. (1962). *The Structure of Scientific Revolutions*. Chicago: University of Chicago Press.

Malan, D.H. (1995). *Individual Psychotherapy and the Science of Psychodynamics*, 2nd edn. Oxford: Butterworth-Heinemann.

Margison, F.R., Loebl, R. and McGrath, G. (1998). 'The Manchester experience: audit and psychotherapy services in northwest England.' In *Rethinking Clinical*

Audit: The Case of Psychotherapy Services in the NHS, eds. R. Davenhill and M. Patrick. London: Routledge.

May, C. (1991). 'Affective neutrality and involvement in nurse–patient relationships: perceptions of appropriate behaviour among nurses in acute medical and surgical wards.' *Journal of Advanced Nursing* 16: 552–8.

Meares, R., Stevenson, J. and Comerford, A. (1999). 'Psychotherapy with borderline patients: a comparison between treated and untreated cohorts.' *Australian and New Zealand Journal of Psychiatry* 33: 467–72.

Menzies I.E.P. (1970). *The Functioning of Social Systems as a Defence Against Anxiety*. London: Tavistock,.

Meutzel, P. (1988). 'Therapeutic nursing.' In *Primary Nursing: Nursing in the Burford and Oxford Nursing Development Unit*, ed. A. Pearson. London: Croom Helm.

Mok, E. and Chiu, P. (2004). 'nurse–patient relationships in palliative care.' *Journal of Advanced Nursing* 48(5): 475–86.

Morrison, E. (1990). 'Violent psychiatric inpatients in a public hospital.' *Scholarly Inquiry for Nursing Practice* 4: 65–82.

Morse, J.M. (1991). 'Negotiating commitment and involvement in the nurse–patient relationship.' *Journal of Advanced Nursing* 16: 455–68.

Morse, J.M. (2006). 'Towards a praxis theory of suffering.' In *The Essential Concepts of Nursing*, eds. J.R. Cutliffe and H.P. McKenna. Edinburgh: Elsevier, Churchill-Livingstone.

Morse, J.M., Bottroff, J., Anderson, G., O'Brien, B. and Solberg, S. (1992). 'Beyond empathy: expanding expressions of caring.' *Journal of Advanced Nursing* 17: 809–21.

Morse, J.M., Bortroff, J., Anderson, G., O'Brien, B. and Solberg, S. (2006). 'Beyond empathy: expanding expressions of caring.' *Journal of Advanced Nursing* 53(1): 75–87.

Moyle, W. (2003). 'Nurse–patient relationship: a dichotomy of expectations.' *International Journal of Mental Health Nursing* 12: 103–9.

National Health Service (NHS) Centre for Reviews and Dissemination (1999). *Effective Health Care: Getting Evidence into Practice. The University of York/NHS Centre for Reviews and Dissemination*. London: The Royal Society of Medicine Press Limited.

O'Kelly, G. (1998). 'Counter transference in the nurse–patient relationship: a review of the literature.' *Journal of Advanced Nursing* 28(2): 391–7.

Odegard, W. (2005). 'Chronic illness as a challenge to the attachment process.' *Clinical Child Psychology and Psychiatry* 10(1): 13–22.

Olsen, D.P. (1997). 'When the patient causes the problem: the effect of patient responsibility on the nurse patient relationship.' *Journal of Advanced Nursing* 26(3): 515–22.

Omdahl, B.L. and O'Donnell, C. (1999). 'Emotional contagion, empathic concern and communicative responsiveness as variables affecting nurses' stress and occupational commitment.' *Journal of Advanced Nursing* 29(6): 1351–67.

Paley, G., Shapiro, D.A., Myers, J., Patrick, S. and Reid, E. (2003). 'Personal reflections of mental health nurse to use the Hobson conversational model (psychodynamic – interpersonal) of psychotherapy.' *Journal of Psychiatric and Mental Health Nursing* 10(6): 735–42.

Payne, N. (2001). 'Occupational stressors and coping as determinants of burnout in female hospice nurses.' *Journal of Advanced Nursing* 33: 396–405.

Payne, S., Dean, S. and Kalus, C. (1998). 'A comparative study of death anxiety in hospice and emergency nurses.' *Journal of Advanced Nursing* 28: 700–6.

Peplau, H.E. (1988). *Interpersonal Relations in Nursing*. London: MacMillan Education Ltd.

Polanyi, M. (1962). *Personal Knowledge*. London: Routledge and Kegan Paul.

Polit, D., Beck, C. and Hungler, B. (2006). *Essentials of Nursing Research: Methods, Appraisal and Utilization*, 4th edn. Philadelphia: JB Lippincott.

Rafferty, M. (2000). 'A conceptual model for clinical supervision in nursing and health visiting based on Winnicott's (1960) theory of the parent infant relationship.' *Journal of Psychiatric and Mental Health Nursing* 7: 153–61.

Ramos, M.C. (1992). 'The nurse–patient relationship: theme and variations.' *Journal of Advanced Nursing* 17: 496–506.

Rasmussen, B.H., Sandman, P. and Norberg, A. (1997). 'Stories of being a hospice nurse: a journey towards finding one's footing.' *Cancer Nursing* 20(5): 330–41.

Richardson, P. (2001). 'Evidence based practice and the psychodynamic psychotherapies.' In *Evidence in the Psychological Therapies – A Practical Guide for Practitioners*, eds. C. Mace, S. Moorey, B. Roberts. Hove and New York: Brunner-Routledge.

Rittman, M., Paige, P., Rivera, J., Sutphin, L., and Godown, I. (1997). 'Phenomenological study of nurses caring for dying patients.' *Cancer Nursing* 20(2): 115–19.

Rodin, G., Walsh, A., Zimmermann, C., Galiese, C., Jones, J., Shepherd, F., Moore, M. Braun, M., Donner, A. and Mikulincer, M. (2007). 'The contribution of attachment security and social support to depressive symptoms in patients with metastatic cancer.' *Psycho-Oncology* 16(12): 1080--91.

Rogers, C. (1951). *Client Centred Therapy*. New York: Houghton Mifflin,

Roth, A. and Fonagy, P. (1996). 'Translating research into practice.' In *What Works for Whom? A Critical Review of Psychotherapy Research*, eds. A. Roth and P. Fonagy. New York: Guilford Press, pp. 13–36.

Rowe, J. (2003). 'The suffering of the healer.' *Nursing Forum* 38(4): 16–20.

Ryecroft-Malone, J., Seers, K., Titchen, A., Harvey, G., Kitson, A. and McCormack, B. (2004). 'What counts as evidence in evidence-based practice?' *Journal of Advanced Nursing* 47(1): 81–90.

Shapiro, D.A., Barkham, M., Rees, A., Hardy, G., Reynolds, S. and Startup, M. (1994). 'Effects of treatment duration and severity of depression on the effectiveness of cognitive-behavioural and psychodynamic-interpersonal psychotherapy.' *Journal of Consulting and Clinical Psychology* 62: 522–34.

Shapiro, D.A., Barkham, M., Rees, A., Hardy, G.E., Reynolds, S. and Startup, M. (1995). 'Decisions, decisions: determining the effect of treatment method and duration on the outcome of psychotherapy for depression.' In *Research Foundations for Psychotherapy Practice*, eds. M. Aveline and D.A. Shapiro. Chichester: Wiley, pp. 151–74.

Skilbeck, J. and Payne, S. (2003). 'Emotional support and the role of clinical nurse specialists in palliative care.' *Journal of Advanced Nursing* 43(5): 521–30.

Storr, A. (2002). *The Art of Psychotherapy*, 2nd edn. Oxford: Arnold.

Strauss, S., Green, M.L. and Bell, D.S. (2004). 'Evaluating the teaching of evidence based medicine: conceptual framework.' *British Medical Journal* 329: 1029–32.

Tellis, W. (1997). 'Introduction to case study.' The Qualitative Report 3(2).

Thompson, S. (1996). 'Empathy: towards a clearer meaning for nursing.' *Nursing Praxis in New Zealand* 11(1): 19–26.

Travelbee, J. (1972). *Interpersonal Aspects of Nursing*. Philadelphia: FA Davis Company.

Turner, M. (2001). *Nurse Involvement and Coping with Cancer Patients*. Unpublished PhD thesis, Kings College University.

Winnicott, D. (1960). 'The theory of the parent-infant relationship.' *International Journal of Psychoanalysis* 41: 585–95.

Wispe, L. (1986). 'The distinction between empathy and sympathy: to call forth a concept, a word is needed.' *Journal of Personality and Social Psychology* 50: 314–21.

Yuen, F.K.H. (1986). 'The nurse-client relationship: a mutual learning experience.' *Journal of Advanced Nursing* 11(4): 529–33.

Chapter 13
'Fevered love'
Alun Jones

Introduction

Later

When you face old age and its natural conclusion
your courage will be shown in little ways,
each spring will be a sword you sharpen,
those you love will live in a fever of love, and you'll bargain with the calendar
and at the last moment
when death opens the back door
you'll put on your carpet slippers
and stride out.

(Anne Sexton, 'Courage', 1975)
Reprinted by permission of SLL/Sterling Lord Literistic Inc. © Anne Sexton

This chapter describes aspects of a research study, which concerned organising a small clinical supervision group made up of five hospice nurses. The study was conducted several years ago. The discussion illustrates ways in which group work might contribute to palliative care, research, education and professional practice more generally. Beneficial factors of group clinical supervision, as experienced by the hospice nurses are also identified. To conclude, the chapter surveys hospice nurses' experiences of professional practice along with the challenges of providing care to the seriously ill, the dying and bereaved. In this study nurses contested with themselves, each other and different professional groups about the finitude of living.

The chapter provides an overview of the research and is directly concerned with the overlaps between professional and personal aspects of living. The study therefore taps into unconscious fundamentals of human existence. It explores some elements of group clinical supervision that hospice nurses found most and least helpful. The concern was with both clinical supervision and groups. In many ways the study replicates tried and tested research methodologies and so cannot lay claim to pioneering status. Nevertheless, the hospice nurses' experiences of small group clinical supervision offer a modest, yet significant contribution to our understanding of beneficial forces operating in clinical supervision groups. Other detailed, yet different accounts of this study are reported elsewhere (Jones, 2003a, 2003b, 2005).

Knowing something about the ways in which clinical supervision can help nurses seems important. We need to know how it works best in order to effectively meet the needs of nurses and enhance clinical practice.

The need for an environment of support and learning

Support and learning

That hospice nursing and palliative care nursing more generally are stressful occupations is well documented, including concerns about providing culturally sensitive care, staff conflict, personal death anxiety and 'burnout' (Ekblad *et al.*, 2000; Jones and Cutcliffe, 2009; Payne *et al.*, 2004). Corner (2002) has written of the many complexities of nurse/patient relationships in palliative care settings. She also discusses nurses' difficulties in communicating with people in their care: likening the effects of working with issues of death and dying to a 'scarring' from war. Nurses working with issues concerning death, dying and bereavement are involved in intense relationships in an area of health care which is commonly considered unpalatable and so difficult to speak about.

Support for workers who provide palliative care therefore seems essential for the safety of the practitioner and quality of care provided. Several documents published in the United Kingdom (Department of Health, 1993; Department of Health, 1994; UKCC, 1996; NMC, 2006) recommend clinical supervision as a means of enhancing the delivery of health care, along with support and continuing education for nurses. Work discussions in clinical supervision could help nurses to understand better the complexities of nursing practice, by learning from their experiences. Skilbeck *et al.* (2005) concur and have suggested that clinical supervision could be helpful to those working in the area of palliative care. Yet they indicate that little is known about the process of clinical supervision or whether it is effective in supporting the work of palliative care. Williamson and Dodds (1999) believe group-format clinical supervision has potential to help nurses but also point to a dearth of evidence for its effectiveness.

Similarly, Lindahl and Norberg (2002) noted that outcomes for clinical supervision groups are not generally reported in the literature. The authors conducted research exploring group-format clinical supervision with enrolled and registered nurses and each group found different gains from clinical supervision. Nevertheless, both groups found that the mutually supportive atmosphere of group clinical supervision allowed members to feel less isolated. Sharing their experiences contributed to better self-management by the nurses and the professional conversations that took place in clinical supervision subsequently benefited nursing care.

An outline of the research study

Outline of the study

This research study was conducted for the reasons given above. What follows is an outline and final report. The project was designed in such a way as to encompass two important areas of professional practice and to attempt to make links between them, namely, supportive supervision of clinical practice and addressing patients' concerns efficiently.

The design of the study acknowledged the demands made on hospice nurses, through daily contact with people suffering serious illness and their families. Group format clinical supervision allowed the hospice nurses time away from the workplace to think about their practice and consider the personal and professional resources needed to carry out their work. Permission to carry out the study was granted by an Ethics Committee, a Hospice Management Team and the nurses involved.

How did the study work?

Essentially, there were two strands woven through this study. The first concerned a small supervision group. We met together in the nurses' workplace, one hour weekly for twelve weeks. Issues concerning professional practice were examined with the help of a researcher (AJ) who acted as the group leader. Group discussions were considered within a psychoanalytical framework, which helped to make sense of sometimes perplexing human dynamics influencing nursing work. At the end of the group's life, nurses were asked by the researcher to complete a questionnaire related to the workplace and to twelve identified therapeutic factors derived from the group experience.

The questionnaire was adapted from an established Q-sort or card scoring system (Yalom, 1975, 1995) intended to identify the most and least helpful factors provided by group experiences. Two weeks later, the hospice nurses were interviewed in a group format and asked to consider the reasons for their choice of answers. This part of the evaluation was carried out sensitively. The study did not appraise individuals but rather the group format of clinical supervision, in its aim of providing an effective learning tool and support for hospice nurses in their day-to-day clinical practice.

Group outcomes

Group outcomes

The data revealed that collectively: *Interpersonal Learning (Output), Identification, Catharsis, Family Re-enactment, Group Cohesiveness* and *Self-understanding* were experienced by the hospice nurses as the most helpful factors of the group. *Existential Factors, Guidance, Universality, Interpersonal Learning (Input), Instillation of Hope* and *Altruism* were identified as less important (see Appendix 1, page 241). Variations in individual responses showed different ways in which a group might meet the needs of its members.

This study was conducted with a small group of committed and motivated hospice nurses who chose to join the group, following a meeting with the researcher. Clinical supervision helped nurses to consider aspects of their professional practice and contribute to their colleagues' practice through listening, thinking about issues and offering opinions. The group tasks focused on collaborative learning, support and the management of care. The second strand was concerned with developing the nurses' competence as listeners, which aimed to enhance their capacity to provide psychological care to their patients.

The clinical supervision group

Clinical supervision group

The group enjoyed excellent working facilities and the encouragement of an enthusiastic and supportive nurse manager. Perhaps unsurprisingly however, the study suggests that working with serious illness, death and bereavement is emotionally demanding of nurses. Nurses in this group shared clinical narratives, which reflected feelings of accomplishment, loss, shame, fear and saturation with issues concerning serious illness, dying and bereavement.

Group members also struggled to make sense of complex human dynamics, which influenced their relationships with both client groups and fellow professionals. Attempts to separate personal concerns from professional issues were, as well, a common and recurring theme throughout the group's life. For example, some nurses spoke about increased death awareness because of their work, causing life in general to seem tasteless and often pointless. Others explained the ways in which anxieties caused by their work spilled over into personal relationships, thereby drawing attention to the high levels of distress invoked in each nurse because of recurrent exposure to distressing situations.

The group nonetheless gave members an experience through which the difficulties concerned with hospice work could be contained and anxieties moderated, through open and frank discussions concerning the challenges of this type of work. The group also offered opportunities for nurses to affirm each other and think about all that was good about their professional practice and their own contributions to providing comfort to patients and families throughout critical times. The group experiences, while initially anxiety-provoking, presented each nurse with opportunities to give and receive support. Group members could feel less isolated, as the following comment demonstrates: 'Being in the group helped me to know a bit more about how the others see me that was helpful. It seemed to help me balance the tempo in and out of work' (Jones, 1999).

The nurses in this study were commanding of respect. Their professional commitment and integrity was praiseworthy, showing at all times concern for their work and their colleagues. Even during periods of negative feelings, the nurses who formed

229

this group wrestled with the appropriateness of their thoughts and behaviours and wanted to carry out all aspects of work to the best of their abilities. The hospice nurses in many instances showed advanced clinical knowledge and expertise concerned with providing physical and psychological pain control. All nurses also demonstrated an unwavering sense of humanity in the face of recurrent challenges and this may be a consequence of the personalities of nurses attracted to this type of work.

'Fevered love'

'Fevered love'

Hospice nurses frequently reported viewing the order of the world as turned upside down, yet they cared deeply about people whose deaths were untimely and without comfort. All nurses spoke about the helplessness they felt recurrently aroused through watching another suffer. Sometimes the people entrusted to their care were colleagues, invoking powerful processes of identification. Several nurses spoke of difficulties caring for people they knew as contemporaries, who had fallen ill.

One nurse spoke of a man she had nursed until death. He had previously been known as a popular colleague and had become physically ill with an infectious illness. She recalled how providing nursing care had been painful for all concerned and how he had been admitted to the hospice for medical and nursing care. The man had lost his sight just before his death and his pain became difficult to check.

The nurse spoke of a collective sense of failing because of the inability to control his pain and a strong sense of helplessness for all, while watching over him. The personal could not be separated from the professional and she conveyed a strong impression of sadness, as she remembered her colleague's illness and progression to death. All nurses spoke of how attempts to provide the consummate death would sometimes prove unsuccessful, causing emotional upheavals within themselves and between colleagues. One example concerned a man who wished to place his face on the tiled floor of his room because it reminded him of home. Nurses spoke of the concern showed by certain members of the team because of such idiosyncratic behaviours, believing that he should remain in bed.

Arguably, the fevered and frenzied attempts to provide a peaceful and a dignified death represent a psychological defence against the reality of death (Deffner and Bell, 2005). Hospice nurses' daily environments are filled with painful experiences and so they bear witness to struggles between living and non-existence. One nurse told of her observations, describing how sometimes people in her care are:

> No longer a part of life nor are they dead. Yet some are a part of one more than the other. Some people though alive are trying to turn to death while others are dying desperately turning to life. Some simply turn their faces to the wall [give themselves up to death]. Sometimes nurses struggle with that and are uncomfortable when a dying person turns his or her face to the wall. (Jones, 1999)

Notions of a timely, consummate and courageous end to life, as reflected in the poem which prefaces this chapter, were therefore challenged almost daily and seemingly influenced nurses' relationships with themselves, colleagues, and families. Nurses were challenged by demands for conformity, and worries could not be left behind in the workplace but were displaced into family situations, that provided apposite but untimely reminders that death permeates life. Working with issues concerning serious illness enhanced a sense of living in an uncertain world. While this could reasonably be considered a human given, nurses who formed the group seemed unable to find relief from the worries of existence.

Nurses in this study referred repeatedly to death as unjust, untimely, and wretched and so were denied a sense of peace, purpose or equanimity, regardless of each nurse's personal effort or commitment. These views perhaps reflect the literature concerning this area of nursing practice (Corner, 2002, Ekblad *et al.*, 2000, Payne *et al.*, 1998). From self reports, it seems cycles of caring in hospice settings are at times compulsive and fast-paced. The nurses used their time in clinical supervision to work together in helpful and supportive ways, *yet all* told of difficulties in sharing their professional experiences with other group members. Although the nurses worked daily as a team, personal affinity could not be assumed.

Nurses and their patients

The hospice nurses nonetheless showed fortitude in recognising and facing difficulties, as a consequence of the clinical supervision group. Each nurse began to set about organising and pacing the delivery of care differently and was less unsettled, as each began to appreciate the difficulties and challenges presented to them by their work. This is captured in the following comments:

> I think that I do this all the time [talk about work] but it is informally and so no change comes from it. This is probably more likely to change my practice. (Jones, 1999)

> I discovered from being in the group things, which I think I already knew yet needed to find the words for. It will change my practice. (Jones, 1999)

Bertman (1991) argues that in Western society, notions of the perfect death often encompass ideas of:

> Timelessness, painlessness, consciousness and prepared-ness. Death would come in later years: it would not be premature. We would be in control of our faculties and alert and able to communicate. The occasion would not occur suddenly but rather eventually with time for both philosophical and emotional preparation. We would be able to speak last words and receive responsive farewells. (Bertman, 1991, p.16)

As Bertman judged, a death, which is both romantic and aesthetic and where communications are regulated and controlled, might rarely be achievable. Yet, this small research study suggested that hospice nurses sometimes feel obliged to make possible the ideal end to life. Subsequently, they become caught up in what the North American poet Anne Sexton referred to in her poem 'Courage' as a 'fever of love', referring to a manic defence mechanism (see Chapter 4). That is to say death should always occur as a loving, peaceful, calm, timely and dignified event and nurses should feel compassion for all in their care without personal consequences. Such unrealistic expectations can lead to high levels of anxiety, with unthought-through activity potentially leading to burn-out.

Work discussions offered through clinical supervision, albeit time-limited and intense, offered some means to nurses of calming the fever and gathering together personal resources. Nurses were better able to regulate emotional responses to challenging situations because of an acknowledgement of the emotional, interpersonally-charged nature of providing end-of-life care. As this nurse states: 'I began to realise [because of the group] that the extraordinary becomes the ordinary and that the effect our work has on us is extraordinary and we need to learn about that' (Jones, 1999).

All nurses spoke about their own feelings in relation to their work, related to hurt, misunderstandings and achievements and again wondered how they might bring about beneficial changes. Every one of the nurses spoke about not being understood and of how less experienced nurses or nursing auxiliaries would seemingly blame them for what might seem an unsatisfactory death. This acknowledgement appeared at a time when all nurses in the group were able to genuinely affirm themselves and each other for their efforts, and could look realistically at the difficulties concerned with hospice work. It was as if they could now allow themselves to use the embedded knowledge gained from their work, and each pondered on how their supervision needs might be fulfilled after the group had ended.

With time, group members became more adept at using the group meetings and we could start to transfer experiential learning from the group to other areas of professional practice. All nurses spoke more freely and it seemed, with greater trust in me as the group leader. One nurse spoke of realising for the first time that when a man in his care wept, in the face of the awfulness of his life situation, there was nothing the nurse could do to prevent the tears of anguish. He told of sitting quietly with the man and offering his presence and understanding. He also told of how he had known this to be helpful from his reading but had just begun to understand fully what it meant to his work. The group, it seemed, was offering to the nurses new, experiential ways of understanding themselves and their work.

This seems to suggest that because of work discussions, the nurse was better able to contain (see Chapters 1 and 2) and moderate anxiety and so be less likely to 'sponge' it up, in an effort to be curative. Positive and beneficial changes had occurred, following our work discussions in supervision. All nurses spoke enthusiastically about making realistic and appropriate changes in the work place and how each individual could improve communication with other staff members, both junior and senior. For example, several nurse spoke of ways in which they assumed responsibility for tasks that could be carried out by other grades of staff and so, as well as feeling burdened with responsibility, they also felt isolated, and denied others opportunities to learn experientially about the work.

I encouraged all nurses to think and share their feelings regarding the end of the group and to think about their supervision or as all preferred to call it, 'work discussion' needs for the future. One nurse told of how, in response to a request for staff support, she organised a work discussion group and spoke of transferring experiences from our small group to the larger setting. A good feeling pervaded our group, with everyone contributing and each supporting another. There seemed to be a sense of constructive hope; we could build an environment in which uncertainty and change were better tolerated.

Learning from one another

Clinical supervision in this study allowed the hospice nurses to learn from each other and about themselves, with reference to their working environment. It also gave all nurses opportunities to offer support and recognise how others value them as fellow workers. The nurses began with tentatively sharing their experiences of professional practice. However, as they became more familiar with group work and began to feel safer with their fellow group members and facilitator, discussions became more vibrant with spontaneous contributions more forthcoming.

The nurses frequently, through their discussions, showed immense personal courage in the face of complex care provision, as well as excellence in the delivery of care to vulnerable groups of people. All demonstrated appropriate concern for the well-being of fellow workers. The opportunities to talk and listen about professional practice seemed to heighten confidence and increase empathy towards each other and other professional groups.

The clinical supervision group also helped to moderate

concerns and anxiety related to the sensitive, yet demanding nature of much of hospice nurses' work. Clinical supervision, therefore, granted a way to ensure some measure of safety and ensure the quality of care delivery. Group-format clinical supervision can offer its members a place to moderate anxieties and establish new patterns of behaviour, as each member becomes ready to think about issues concerning professional practice. Reflection before, in, and after clinical practice is shown to be possible and to the benefit of all concerned (Schön, 1983).

Clinical supervision, it seems, can offer occasions for nurses to face themselves and others candidly in relation to their work. A supervisor can be supportive in recognising that psychological defences are necessary for nurses to cope with and survive the demands of hospice work. Hospice nurses can then be helped to understand the complexity of feelings aroused because of their work, which whenever necessary could be restructured, refined or calibrated to show sensitivity and compassion to themselves and others.

To illustrate, one nurse commented that she had recognised as we spoke that, although the hospice nurse's role was concerned with the management of illness, dying and bereavement, she and her colleagues frequently felt that it was their responsibility to address and mend the totality of a person's life. She went on to tell of how this belief aroused feelings of ownership of a person but ultimately resulted in failure, because of the intractable nature of many people's life difficulties (Jones, 1999). All spoke of the dilemmas each experienced through managing their relationships with 'niceness' to patients and families and realised that each felt trapped into being always nice and so disabled or prevented from asserting their needs with others.

Another feature of this study concerns ways in which the group-experience aroused in all nurses issues related to their personal life. A psychodynamic way of thinking allowed each to make meaningful connections with life events that influenced their experiences of the workplace. This seemingly suggests that clinical supervision can be a therapeutic experience for nurses and that the personal cannot be separated from the professional. The emotional wounding and subsequent 'scarring' described by Corner (2002) may however, be prevented or at least minimised. This small, exploratory research study suggested that supervision could provide hospice nurses with time for contemplative, strategic and anticipatory ways of thinking. Nurses can, together and with support, witness the difficulties and challenges of being with others authentically, at times of pain.

Notwithstanding potential benefits, this study also suggests that, initially, group work can arouse anxiety in all participants and preparation and support are required for the group leader and group members. For example, it is important that all concerned have some understanding about likely group processes and the conduct required for successful group membership. Carefully chosen membership is also considered important for the safety of members and success of the group, as the ability to contribute to discussion is critical to good group-outcomes. Furthermore, issues of gender and ethnicity should be considered important to the safety and sensitivity of the group members. There is potential for negative group processes to operate outside of the group member's awareness, leading to projection, scapegoating or the marginalisation of individual group members, to the detriment of all concerned (Kocijan Lovko et al., 2007). Work discussions in the form of clinical supervision meetings are also likely to be helpful to the group facilitator.

So what has been learnt now the research study is completed?

What has been learnt?

The study showed that, with thought, it is possible to establish group, clinical supervision for hospice nurses and identify the potential benefits to be derived from these work discussions. The nurses that formed this group were all courageous and committed health practitioners. They demonstrated the ability to address with sensitivity, complex and frequently poignant issues concerning serious illness, dying and bereavement.

The facilities on hand were excellent and the empathic support from the hospice management team formed a feature of this work. Clinical supervision, or other forms of work discussion, should continue to support the work of hospice nurses and other workers, allowing nurses to manage care, understand better the interpersonal dynamics involved and to disentangle the complexity of emotional work.

This study indicates that there are benefits to be gained from thinking carefully about professional practice. Clinical supervision should form a part of working time, which is protected from the intrusion of other responsibilities. Hospice nurses should undertake further education and training, learning how to become supervisors and be supervised. Perhaps hospices might develop a directory of supervisors, so that nurses could supervise individuals and small groups outside their own work environment.

A noteworthy feature of the group interview that completed the research was the ease with which we were able to discuss issues concerning work and the group experience. Reflecting back to more difficult discussions in the group, I asked the nurses why this might be. All agreed that it was because they knew me better. This might suggest that staying together through difficulties benefits nurses' relationships in supervision. We looked back to our conversations and one nurse told me about a patient's death. I sensed fleeting sorrow within the group, concerning another loss but also perhaps relating to the end of the group's life. I enjoyed our time together and I was sad to say goodbye to respected colleagues. Yet perhaps in contradiction, this also seemed to me a point at which we were potentially at the beginning of something new. The nurses had arranged to continue with clinical supervision, with an invited professional leading the group.

Death awareness

Death awareness

An important aspect of this research study and one frequently overlooked in the literature concerned the emotional impact on me as a group leader. I noted my own awareness of death and sensitivity to life changed during the study. I would dream of issues related to endings and death and my own mortality. I began to think more deeply about meanings and purpose concerning living, so mirroring events as told by the hospice nurses. It was as if, simply by being close to the group, I had unwittingly absorbed the nurses' concerns about life and death and perhaps some that they had assimilated from patients and families in the form of what was referred to by Searles (1955) as a 'parallel process'. This is an emotional process in which feelings can be passed on unconsciously from one person to another, influencing their perceptions of relationships in different ways. The use of the defence mechanism of projective identification (see Chapter 4) creates this phenomenon of parallel process.

Limitations

Limitations

Qualitative research has much to offer to our understanding of health care. However, it is important to be mindful of limitations. With regard to this small study, a single group was used. Also, the purposive research sample and a single male facilitator, who also acted as the researcher, needs to be considered in terms of bias, which influences all interpretive work. Using a non-validated questionnaire might also influence the validity of self reports. Consequently, recommendations cannot be made beyond the context of the study group, as the findings might not relate to all hospice nurses equally. Inferences may be drawn from the study however, and the findings reported in several papers related to this study could offer guidance regarding how clinical supervision might benefit hospice nurses and others concerned with the provision of care to the seriously ill and their families (Jones, 2003a, 2003b, 2006).

Conclusion

> Next, my kinsman, you powdered your sorrow,
> you gave it a back rub
> and then you covered it with a blanket
> and after it had slept a while
> it woke to the wings of the roses
> and was transformed.
>
> *(Anne Sexton, 'Courage', 1975*
> Reprinted by permission of SLL/Sterling Lord Literistic Inc. © Anne Sexton

The chapter concludes by suggesting that clinical supervision, conducted as work discussion groups, can offer hospice nurses the means to compose, regulate and plan their interactions with each other and others. Anne Sexton's poem 'Courage' is essentially about facing up to adversity and so speaks to human 'givens' such as isolation, death and seeking out meaning to life. It is perhaps, in part, because of the courage of hospice nurses, that calm and order is brought to the lives and deaths of many patients and families in times of life crisis.

Accounts of professional practice reported in this research study also suggest that a psychodynamic awareness concerning providing health care to patients in situations of serious illness, dying and bereavement can enhance our understanding of ways anxiety can influence behaviours in various and complex ways.

Hospice care is rooted in a fundamental principle that the seriously ill, the dying and the bereaved require environments characterised by dignity, security and calm. Psychoanalytically informed work discussions, taking place in clinical supervision could go some way to offering similar conditions to hospice nurses. In turn, hospice nurses may be better able to sustain periods of uncertainty and ambiguity, recognise personal and professional influences on care and so be more able to think critically and constructively about themselves. In doing so, they might be helped to meet sensitively, the needs of vulnerable patients and their families.

References

Bertman, S. (1991). *Facing Death*. New York: Hemisphere.

Corner, J. (2002). 'Nurses' experiences of cancer.' *European Journal of Cancer Care* 11(3): 193–9.

Deffner, J.M. and Bell, S.K. (2005). 'Nurses' death anxiety, comfort level during communication with patients and families regarding death, and exposure to communication education: a quantitative study.' Journal for Nurses in Staff Development 21(1): 19–23.

Department of Health (1993). *A Vision for the Future: The Nursing, Midwifery and Health Visiting Contribution to Health and Health Care*. London: HMSO.

Department of Health (1994). 'Clinical supervision; for the nursing and health visiting professions.' *CNO Professional Letter* 94(5), 11 February, London.

Ekblad, S., Marttila, A. and Emilsson, M. (2000). 'Cultural challenges in end-of-life care: reflections from focus groups' interviews with hospice staff in Stockholm.' *Journal of Advanced Nursing* 31(3): 623–30.

Jones, A. (1999). *Fevered Love: an Exploratory Study to Identify Beneficial Factors Experienced by Hospice Nurse Members of a Group Format of Clinical Supervision*. MSc Dissertation, University of Middlesex, unpublished.

Jones, A. (2003a). 'Some benefits experienced by hospice nurses from group clinical supervision.' *European Journal of Cancer Care* 12: 234–72.

Jones, A. (2003b). 'On projective identification, containment and feeling special: some thoughts about hospice nurses' experiences.' *American Journal of Hospice and Palliative Care* 20(6): 441–6.

Jones, A. (2005). 'Group-format clinical supervision for hospice nurses.' *European Journal of Cancer Care* 15(2): 155—62

Jones, A. and Cutcliffe, J.R. (2009). Listening as a method of addressing psychological distress. *Journal of Nursing Management* 17(3): 352–358.

Kocijan Lovko, S., Gregurek, R.E. and Karlovic, D. (2007). 'Stress and ego-defense mechanisms in medical staff at oncology and physical medicine departments.' *European Journal of Psychiatry* 21(4): 279–86.

Lindahl, B. and Norberg, A. (2002). 'Clinical group supervision in an intensive care unit: a space for relief, and for sharing emotions and experiences of care.' *Journal of Clinical Nursing* 11(6): 809–18.

Nursing and Midwifery Council (NMC) (2006). *Clinical Supervision.* http://www.nmc-uk.org/cms/content/Advice/Clinical Supervision. (Accessed 2008)

Payne, S.A., Dean, S.J. and Kalus, C. (1998). 'A comparative study of death anxiety in hospice and emergency nurses.' *Journal of Advanced Nursing* 28(4): 700–6.

Schön, D. (1983). *The Reflective Practitioner: How Professionals Think in Action.* London: Basic Books.

Searles, H. (1955). 'The informational value of the supervisor's emotional experience.' *Psychiatry* 18(4): 135–46.

Sexton, A. (1975). *Courage in the Awful Rowing Toward God.* Boston: Houghton Mifflin Co .Reprinted by permission of SLL/Sterling Lord Literistic Inc.

Skilbeck, J.K., Payne, S.A., Ingleton, M.C., Nolan, M., Carey, I. and Hanson, A.(2005). 'An exploration of family carers' experience of respite services in one specialist palliative care unit.' *Palliative Medicine* 19(8): 610–18.

Williamson, R. and Dodds, S. (1999). 'The effectiveness of a group approach to clinical supervision in reducing stress: a review of the literature.' *Journal of Clinical Nursing* 8(4): 338–44.

Yalom, I.V. (1975). *The Theory and Practice of Group Psychotherapy.* New York: Basic Books.

Yalom, I.V. (1995). *The Theory and Practice of Group Psychotherapy*, 4th edn. New York: Basic Books.

United Kingdom Central Council for Nursing Midwifery and Health Visiting (UKCC) (1996). *Clinical Supervision: Guidelines for Practice.* London: UKCC.

Appendix I

(derived from Yalom 1975 and 1995)

Beneficial Factors

The hospice nurses found the following to be most helpful factors:

- Interpersonal Learning (Output) – Learning about oneself from others.
- Identification – Modelling beneficial behaviours on others.
- Catharsis – getting things off one's chest.
- Family re-enactment – Recognising that groups can sometimes remind us of our family of origin and so current behaviours might derive from past learning.
- Group cohesiveness – Viewing the group as together with common goals.
- Self-understanding – Learning about oneself from the group experience.

The hospice nurses experienced the following factors as less important:

- Existential factors – Factors to do with living in the world and being human: making decisions and accepting responsibilities.
- Guidance – Learning from others' knowledge and experience including feeling supported by the group.
- Universality – Feelings of all being together, or in the same boat.
- Interpersonal Learning (Input) – Learning about how you relate to others.
- Instillation of Hope – Inspiring realistic and constructive feelings that something worthwhile will happen.
- Altruism – Offering or receiving care and guidance to or from others in the group.

Chapter 14
Using Winnicott (1960) to create a model for clinical supervision[2]

Mic Rafferty

In what follows use of the term 'nurse' is generic, applying to all nursing sub-groups.

Introduction

When writing about clinical supervision, a number of authors (Swain, 1995, Winship, 1995, Hughes and Pengelly, 1997) have employed Winnicott's (1960) concept of *holding* to suggest a feature of the supervisory relationship. *Holding* is the ability to have an empathic concern for the supervisee, along with the capacity to provide the conditions for safe supervisory work, to enable appropriate growth and change. Here Winnicott's concept of the 'good enough mother', which refers to the parental need to provide adequate care and concern for the child, helps us to consider the nature of the 'facilitating environment' in clinical supervision. Similar to Winnicott's notion of 'good enough' parental care, perfection is not the expectation of the supervisor. The aim is to provide 'enough holding and containment for confidence and trust to be established' (Swain, 1995, p. 43). Winship's (1995, p. 228) account of clinical supervision with mental health nurses working with acutely disturbed patients finds that to 'hold the patient in their distress' nurses 'need some form of supervisory holding in order that they may process their subjective experience'.

However, when Hughes and Pengelly (1997, p. 178), refer to Winnicott's (1960) 'sense of being held' to convey the importance

[2]This is a revised version of the following article: Rafferty, M.A. (2000). 'A conceptual model for clinical supervision in nursing and health visiting based upon Winnicott's (1960) theory of the parent-infant relationship.' Journal of Psychiatric and Mental Health Nursing 7: 153—61.

in clinical supervision of 'consistency, regularity, clear boundaries and minimising intrusion', they are describing a more complex schema than just *holding*. They draw attention to the need to explain the other dimensions of the facilitating relationship, which are, *handling* and *object presenting*.

A starting point to applying Winnicott's parental ideas to clinical supervision would see *holding* as active, empathic concern for the professional health and welfare of one's colleagues, which leads to a defined relationship based on mutual trust. *Holding* extends into the concept of *handling*, through its requirement to identify the necessary conditions for professional development, and provide opportunities for finding useful meaning in the challenges of change and loss. The creation of such conditions for professional growth has then the potential for a relationship centred on *object presenting*. This involves mutuality, a furthering of professional self-belief and thus the ability for the supervisee to be independent and the author of acts of good, for self and others. The aim of this chapter is to explore Winnicott's theory of the parent–infant relationship and reveal a relevant conceptual framework to understand and guide the process of clinical supervision in nursing. The use of a theory about child-parent relationships as a means of explaining the needs and experiences of adults in clinical supervision is controversial. However, the intention is to demonstrate how such ideas are valuable when illustrating and explaining supervisory process.

The concepts of 'holding', 'handling' and 'object presenting'

The concepts

Winnicott's observations of early infant–maternal relationships drew attention to the 'importance of personal and environmental influences in the development of the individual' (Winnicott, 1960, p. 585). Maternal provision, according to Winnicott:

> protects from physiological insult ... by taking account of the infant's sensitivity to touch, temperature, sound and light, falling and lack of knowledge of the existence of anything other than the self. (Winnicott, 1960, p. 587)

Using Winnicott (1960)

He identified three ways in which the mother protects, orientates and enables the baby to learn from experience and so gain control progressively over self and environment. That is by *holding, handling* and *object presenting* (see Box 14.1).

Box 14.1

The concepts of *Holding, Handling* and *Object Presenting*

HOLDING

Maternal holding is a physical and an emotional act. The 'good-enough mother,' contains and manages her baby's feelings and impulses by empathy, leading her to protect him from too many jarring experiences. Her protective holding is the way she carries, feeds, speaks and responds to her baby, in her understanding of his experience and needs.

HANDLING

This aspect of the early relationship arises from the mother's handling. At its best, her sensitive touch and responsive care of the baby's body, enables him to experience physical and emotional satisfaction in an integrated way. This helps the baby to bring together the worlds of sensation and emotion and begin to build a stable unity of mind and body. An individual who has received sensitive handling in early life will experience his mental, emotional and physical capacities as connected, personal and authentic.

OBJECT PRESENTING

Object presenting is the way in which the mother brings the outside world to her baby. When all goes well, the baby is ready to receive and explore and the mother is happy to allow him some independence. By presenting objects and experiences in a way, which is sensitive to her baby's state, the mother helps him build a primitive conviction of omnipotence, including the ability to be the author of his own success. Thus, the baby develops a sense of oneness and trust in the world, which grows into an appreciation of both his connection with others and his separateness. Therefore, he gains confidence in his ability to reach out and to make changes in the world and expects to meet with understanding and responsiveness.

Adapted from Gomez (1997, pp. 89–90)

'Holding' and clinical supervision

An advantage of Winnicott's theory to inform supervisory practice is that because of its preoccupation with the facilitating environment, its primary concern is with growth, development and the conditions within which these occur, hence mirroring the intended process of clinical supervision. Therefore, it is relevant to

'Holding' and clinical supervision

associate Winnicott's ideas with meeting the ordinary and healthy needs of nurses.

Clinical supervision has maternal aspects as the activity involves containing and managing the feelings and impulses of the supervisee, through demonstrating empathy and protecting the supervisee from the effects of too many 'jarring experiences' (Gomez, 1997). The presence of jarring experiences in care work is increasingly recognised. As was vividly described in Chapter 8, caring for individuals with dementia can engender feelings of meaninglessness, helplessness and anxiety (Hallberg and Norberg, 1993). Lawler (1991) suggests general nurses find it very difficult to talk about their work with non-nurses, as it involves aspects of life considered dirty or too sexual for others' comfort. Smith's (1992) narrative of the care experiences of student nurses points to the unbearable dissonance that can exist between institutional expectations of how nurses should behave and their ordinary impulses. Adams (1996) found loneliness featured in the work experience of community psychiatric nurses. Palsson *et al.*'s (1994) analysis of clinical supervision narratives of district nurses showed they were troubled by coming too close to the patient, keeping and restoring patients' hope, feeling powerless and feelings of disgust, shame and guilt (Palsson *et al.*, 1994). Severinsson (1995) found, during clinical supervision of psychiatric nurses, that significant emotional states existed, involving feelings of guilt about care and work relationships and that these feelings negatively influenced job satisfaction and the ability to develop professionally. Snelgrove's (1998) comparative study of the occupational stress levels experienced by health visitors, district nurses and community psychiatric nurses, generated findings suggesting that job stress factors include: emotional involvement, unpredictable work events and instability surrounding the work content.

Clearly, jarring experiences in professional care are varied and somewhat client-group specific, but they remain poorly understood in terms of their exact manifestation in specific practice areas (McVicar, 2003). Such experiences are used to justify the development of clinical supervision as a vehicle for creative and supportive professional relationships, as it offers the means to articulate the unique stressors of each environment.

Given such illustrations it is possible to see why the case-for an emotional support system (Hallberg 1994) has led to acceptance that clinical supervision should provide support and restoration (Proctor, 1987). Such thinking is in tune with the notion of holding and empathic interest in the work of the supervisee. However, there are problems in accepting that clinical supervision is just an unconditional empathic activity, by which the supervisee is to be relieved of the emotional strain of their work (Hallberg 1994). This, according to Hughes and Pengelly (1997), would suggest that clinical supervision involves 'unconditional positive regard', which risks making support the principal function of clinical supervision, with a loss of emphasis upon ensuring and promoting safe and higher standards of care.

A related issue is the relative reticence in nursing concerning the emotions engendered by caring. From a psychoanalytical perspective, intimate care can expose the nurse to the patient's libidinal and aggressive impulses as well as their own (Fabricius, 1991). Work with ill patients constantly confronts nurses with severe, often life-threatening illness and with death. As a result, nurses have to struggle with anxieties about illness, death, dying, loss, guilt and helplessness (Skogstad, 1997).

Social systems traditionally employed to deal with emotionality in the work place, have relied upon the processes of psychosocial distancing, task allocation, the depersonalisation of patients (Menzies, 1959) and denial, splitting and projective identification (Dartington, 1993). The adoption of a process of clinical supervision, which attends to the emotional world of the worker, means that nursing has to develop ways of learning emotionally from such predicaments.

That such emotional learning is necessary is increasingly recognised in Trust policies about clinical supervision. For instance City and Hackney Teaching Primary Care Trust (2006) acknowledges 'that health professionals are in stressful occupations and therefore do require active support'. This aims 'to provide relief from the emotional and personal stresses involved in nursing' (Worcestershire NHS Mental Health Partnership, 2005). According to Yegdich and Cushing (1998), the UK is unknowingly re-enacting the debate about the purpose of clinical supervision, which has preoccupied psychoanalysis since inception of the practice in the 1920 and 1930s. That is, is its primary purpose 'treating or teaching'? A Winnicottian perspective helps to establish a useful position on this question, by suggesting a way to work with emotions. Such a perspective centres on the belief that the human, inherited tendencies for growth will always reassert themselves, given the right conditions (Phillips, 1988). Clinical supervision would therefore be a growth-orientated relationship process, concerned with learning in the broadest sense. This avoids turning the emotional world of practice into a source of pathology or dysfunction, allowing the emotions engendered by care to be of use in revealing intuitive knowing and so be a means of learning from practice.

Winnicott's notion of maternal containment helps identify the ways in which the supervisor works with the emotions of care. Palsson *et al.* (1994) employ the term 'overwhelming situations' to convey the nurses' sense of not knowing what to do, which was a feature of their narratives brought to clinical supervision. Butterworth *et al.*'s (1997) extracts from clinical supervision provide other examples of emotional states of doubt, with supervisees unable to make useful sense of such experiences. For instance, a nurse presented herself as 'feeling incompetent and guilty of poor judgement'; another had to deal with the fact that 'a patient set fire to themselves'. Another nurse who had 'a family member diagnosed with cancer' found this negatively impacted upon her ability to care for patients with cancer.

In clinical supervision practice, the supervisors of these nurses demonstrated containment by hearing with empathy the overwhelming experience of the supervisee and then enabling the discovery of a tolerable and understandable meaning. Supervisory containment is about helping the supervisee to 'name' an emotional experience in order that they can mobilise appropriate defences to a situation which is 'wrong, painful or downright unbearable' (Dartington, 1993, p. 34) and then be helped to protect themselves from stress, in order that the care task is protected.

A link here is to Winnicott's notion of 'unintegration' (Gomez, 1997). For the infant this is a state of being which either produces senses of being real and comfortable or unreal, ill at ease and at odds with the world. What makes the difference is how the mother manages the maternal environment to ensure its quality is such that the infant is able to manage without being jarred, over-excited or frightened, thus avoiding the baby 'withdrawing' as a means of self-protection. Where maternal care is 'good enough', threats to the infant's sense of self are managed, leading to a state of 'unintegration', enabling the infant to experience a relaxed and undefended openness to the world of experience. Such states make it possible for the infant to develop a sense of true self, based upon experiences which have coherence, continuity and novelty.

In the literature related to clinical supervision in nursing, it is possible to determine a call for an adult equivalent of such a provision, with the hope of similar beneficial consequences for the nurse. A study of the practice of clinical supervision (Rafferty *et al.*, 1998) suggests that an appropriate environment for clinical supervision had characteristics of comfort, privacy and reasonable control of distractions. Palsson *et al.*'s (1994) work revealed that nurses valued the undisturbed analysing of situations. Ritter *et al.*'s (1996) settings for clinical supervision 'ensured psychological and physical safety and comfort'. Some literature calls for a process, which implies 'a relaxed and undefended openness to the world of experience'. For instance, Winship's (1995) supervisees brought their work-related dreams to clinical supervision. Part of Hallberg's (1994, p. 46) process included 'free association to key words'. McCormack and Hopkins (1995, p. 164) worked toward creating a reflective milieu, which was both consistent and spontaneous. Jones' (1997, p. 241) supervision of work with a dying client provided 'creative holding conditions'. Dudley and Butterworth's (1994, p. 39) supervisees valued the 'interplay' that occurred as part of the interaction in clinical supervision. Such examples support the value of a helpful unintegrative (relaxed, spontaneous and unguarded) milieu for clinical supervision.

Clinical supervision has to be concerned with the 'here and now' work of the supervisee. Based on the limited descriptions available, issues raised are often about professional anxieties (Bishop, 1998) and demanding interpersonal issues (Rafferty, 1999). Use of Winnicott's (1960) notions of maternal provision to aid thinking about clinical supervision helps keep in mind that 'when it goes well', it does not lead to the 'closing down' of the supervisee, but rather to a state of creative play. This enables sensations and ideas about practice to develop into a tangible, useful form, leading to an enhanced ability to be the author of our own and others' good.

Nurses and their patients

The literature about clinical supervision consistently points to the qualities the supervisor will need to bring to the relationship (Faugier, 1992a, Chambers and Long, 1995, Jones, 1996, Jansson and Norberg, 1993). From the idealistic to the realistic, many of the qualities listed by these authors are relationship skills, supporting Jones' (1996) claim that relationship quality is of greater significance than issues of method. Winnicott's thinking not only helps us to keep a sense of proportion (supervisory care aims to be 'good enough' not perfect) but also aids recognition of the importance of the supervisor responding appropriately to the unique needs of the supervisee. This suggests that the level of the supervisor's preoccupation with the needs of the supervisee varies at different points in their supervisee's professional development.

Arguably, supervisor preoccupation with the needs of the supervisee establishes the conditions for a supervisor to become an 'attachment figure' (Bowlby, 1988). Attachment theory suggest that 'all of us, from the cradle to the grave, are happiest when life is organised as a series of excursions, long or short, from the secure base provided by our attachment figures' (Bowlby, 1988, p. 62).

The everydayness and importance of work attachment behaviour is observable in an effective ward team, which can display moods of fondness, liking, mutuality, and so called team spirit and teamwork. One aims to replicate this attachment spirit within the clinical supervision relationship, both one to one and group, though with one important difference. Given that a consequence of such worker mutuality can be like-mindedness, it is increasingly recognised that effective supervision is more likely to occur if the relationship is created outside usual team and hierarchical relationships (Winstanley, 2001), thereby creating the conditions for peer attachments, which have the potential for novel ways of thinking, because the perspectives of others from different care systems make it more possible to explore the world of practice.

Winnicott's concept of maternal holding has been used to make a developmental case for nurses to have helpful 'unintegrative' experiences, which enable them to make sense of threats to their self, so they remain authentic to themselves and their profession. *Holding* is central to the supportive-restorative function of clinical supervision and the legitimate need to have professional attachment figures.

'Handling' and clinical supervision

For Winnicott, sensitive and responsive body care allows the baby to establish a stable integration and unity out of the worlds of sensation (the feelings of the body) and thinking (the images of the mind), that is, to establish a 'psychosomatic relationship' (Gomez, 1997) between the body and its responses and the developing mental images of self and the world.

In this context, Butterworth *et al.*'s (1997) evaluative research of clinical supervision in England and Scotland, advised nursing to take a particular interest in psychosomatic issues. They determined clear associations between how individuals estimated their personal physical fitness and their psychological well-being, with sickness and absence lower when respondents reported better fitness levels. However, no explanation is given or link made with the work environment to explain this phenomenon, just a recommendation that employers 'encourage' the pursuit of healthy lifestyles by their workers (Butterworth *et al.*, 1997). More might have been made then of the finding that nurses never had so much work stress. Work-related stress can be sufficiently serious to put patients at risk and is implicated in the development of the extreme condition of 'burn out' (Mimura and Griffiths, 2003). A study of ward sisters by Allen (2001) determined that much of their stress originated from organisational and managerial factors, which they felt to be beyond their control. They report their roles becoming increasingly complex, with additional responsibilities heaped upon them. With management imperatives and targets imposed and with insufficient consultation or consideration about their implementation, the ward sisters found it very difficult to get their voices heard (Allen, 2001). A survey by the *Nursing Times* magazine (2007) of almost 2,000 nurses, found seventy per cent said they suffered from physical or mental health problems linked to work-related stress. Forty-four per cent said their sex life was suffering as a result and a quarter said they had started drinking more. The poll also found one in ten nurses were smoking more, and almost a third reported taking off more days sick than usual.

Many reports by nurses during educational preparation for clinical supervision (Rafferty, 1999) left the impression that nursing work practices (particularly in acute care) led to unhealthy behaviours. The customary nursing defence of stoicism (displayed particularly by senior nurses) seemed to have led to a norm of missed breaks and meals, lengthy spans of duty, duty changes at short notice and the frequent taking of administrative work home for completion. More recently, the Royal College of Nursing (2008b) determined that the annual employment figures for Wales showed that nurses did on average more than four hours unpaid work every week.

Wolsey and Leach (1997, p. 25) suggest it is important to accept that: '45 minutes per month of even world class supervision is unlikely to be enough to help people who may spend the remaining 149 hours ... in hostile working environments'. However, when clinical supervision is established as an orientating rhythm or customary practice, it provides a reference point for bringing the mind and body experiences of the world of work together. This is necessary in order to help nurses determine 'good enough' responses to demands from others (health/educational organisations) which have implications for their body (physical demands) and their mind (competency demands).

Handling has relevance to the management and delivery of clinical supervision. The literature would suggest that delivery issues have to do with structure (Bodley, 1992) and authority (UKCC, 1996). In the early maternal relationship, it is the mother, through understanding the infant's developmental needs, who determines the form of *handling*. She has the power to determine the form of delivery of her care, though society is quick to call her to account for abuse of such power. In current thinking about clinical supervision, there is no such clarity about when it might be developmentally appropriate for the supervisor to have the ability to limit or stop another's practice. This perhaps results from widespread worries that clinical supervision will take on the ethos of managerial supervision. Jones (1996) suggests the 'literature reads like a litany of fears ... that supervision will become contaminated with overseeing, directional and inspective functions' (Jones, 1996, p. 291). Such anxieties about managerial supervision should not be allowed to undermine the exercise of appropriate professional authority in clinical supervision. For as identified by Rafferty and Coleman (1996) effective clinical supervision involves the exercise of appropriate authority. Failure to see that clinical supervision involves authority of purpose and therefore the potential for appropriate limit setting, could reduce clinical supervision to a series of isolated, unaccountable, undirected and under-resourced interactions.

The principal purpose of maternal *handling* is to provide the baby with a sense of connection and orientation to his body and his world. Failure of such a provision can leave the child with an incomplete idea about what is up or down, inside or out, forwards or backwards, with the ability to connect together what he feels and thinks is right or wrong compromised. The mother, through her monitoring and responses, makes decisions about what to 'fuss about or not fuss about' (Winnicott, 1988) thereby supporting the infant's orientation towards what is mentally or physically significant or important. The failure to provide secure maternal *handling* is linked to the development of an anti-social tendency (Gomez, 1997). Therefore, it should be a concern of any caring discipline to ensure that its practitioners have the ability to act in ways which are congruent with what they feel and think, within the boundaries of acceptable professional conduct. Clinical supervision can provide regular opportunities for such an orientation to be realised.

How this monitoring or normative function for clinical supervision is actualised causes concern. For while there is a widely held conviction that what to 'fuss about' should not be driven by organisational or hierarchical priorities, with a professional agenda for monitoring preferred, none of the professional infrastructure, unlike midwifery (NMC, 2008b) is available to nursing (NMC, 2008a).

A widely accepted (NMC, 2008b, NHS Scotland, 2008.) professional orientation for the handling work of clinical supervision is available in the NHS Management Executive (Department of Health, 1993) definition of clinical supervision. This views clinical supervision as:

> ... a formal process of professional support and learning, which enables individual practitioners to develop knowledge and competence, assume responsibility for their own practice and enhance consumer protection and safety of care in complex situations.
>
> (Department of Health, 1993)

The task is to translate this orientation into patterns of supervisory *handling* within which it is possible to both feel and think about the characteristics of safe and appropriate professional practice, in complex situations.

Attention to the handling dimensions of time for and frequency of clinical supervision (Butterworth *et al.*, 1997, Jenkins *et al.*, 2000, Rafferty *et al.*, 2007) suggests that a pragmatic, as opposed to a theoretical understanding, is driving the implementation of clinical supervision. As Jones (1996) points out, creating an environment conducive to the contemplation of practice, which employs clinical supervision, will have daunting resource implications. For instance, Butterworth *et al.*'s (1997) study was compromised by practitioners' inability to meet the time requirements for clinical supervision. Much has changed since Bishop's report (1998) that many Trust executive nurses, while supportive of clinical supervision, could take it no further than pilot projects because of 'the lack of a costing model which could be set against hard outcomes'(Bishop, 1998, p. 148). Clinical supervision is regarded now as an important part of clinical governance (NMC 2008), with some Trusts now regarding clinical supervision as a necessary mandatory practice by their nursing staff (Abbott *et al.*, 2006). It still seems, though, that while theoretical explanations can tell us something of the *handling* process, for example, how to talk (Faugier, 1992b), a convincing, overarching conceptual framework has not been established, which could make it an imperative to provide clinical supervision within an established period of time. For instance, Trust recommendations about the necessary frequency of clinical supervision can range from no recommended frequency (Dudley Group of Hospitals, 2004) to a maximum of every two months with a three monthly minimum requirement (Leicester County and Rutland NHS Primary Care Trust, 2006). Salisbury Health Care Trust (2004) recommends that clinical supervision sessions should last for approximately one hour and take place monthly.

Returning to the orientating principle for clinical supervision provided by NHS Management Executive (DoH, 1993), it could be argued that the function of *handling* in clinical supervision is to produce developmentally appropriate professional change. For to 'develop knowledge and competence' is overtly about change, and to 'assume responsibility for their own practice' and 'enhance consumer protection and safety of care in complex situations' implies the need to question what we do. Change processes are difficult. In the growth of infants, which is driven by a powerful biological imperative, it is possible to show that they get stuck when forced to deal with upsetting or unpredictable events, without a secure relationship within which it is possible to 'protest, adapt and/or mourn' (Hughes and Pengelly, 1997, p. 136). The work of Marris (1986) suggests a similar process is observable in studies of how adults cope and adapt in situations of loss and change. Therefore the *handling* dimension in clinical supervision has to be frequent enough to meet human needs for protest and for determining meaning, followed by time for adaptation and/or mourning, all within the context of delivering 'good enough' care.

'Object presenting' and clinical supervision

'Object presenting' and clinical supervision

Object presenting refers to the ways the mother brings the outside world to the baby. The development of reciprocity between the infant and the mother facilitates the baby's instinctual abilities to both receive and explore. Maternal attunement by 'good enough' responsiveness to the infant's exploratory drive provides an experience, which is neither too quick nor too slow. When 'all goes well' the baby develops an ability to associate his responses with a desirable outcome. So begins the infant's belief in his capacity to bring about change through his own actions.

With regard to clinical supervision and adults, it is possible to suggest that the literature is calling for something similar to maternal responsiveness in the supervisor and in the nature of organisational support. For instance, the best kind of organisational arrangements will 'develop process relevant to local circumstances' and what registered nurses see as needed (NMC, 2008a). The literature drives home the idea that clinical supervision has to be led by the interests, excitements and concerns of the supervisee (Faugier, 1992a, Morton-Cooper and Palmer, 1993, Chambers and Long, 1995, Titchen and Binnie, 1995, Ritter *et al.*, 1996). That clinical supervision is a reciprocal relationship is consistently identified, although expressed in terms such as 'exchange' (Butterworth *et al.*, 1996), 'sharing' (Dudley and Butterworth, 1994), 'collegial'

(McCormack and Hopkins, 1995) or 'mutual' (Jones, 1996).

The reciprocity, which the mother–child couple have to achieve in order to feed successfully, suggests that the restorative and learning functions of clinical supervision are more likely to be met in reciprocal conditions and that such functions are congruent with the essential nature of nursing, which is to nurture (Nightingale, 1860, Peplau, 1988). It has been argued that nurture is an inadequate concept to capture the purpose of clinical supervision, as it is supposedly not about enabling and affirming (Morcom and Hughes, 1996). However Inskipp and Proctor's (1993, p. 6) definitions of supervisory restoration and learning are capable of being understood within the concept of maternal nurture. They include: 'the provision of space', 'the chance to explore opportunities', 'discharging held emotions', 'recharging energies, ideals and creativity' and 'shared responsibility for ... development in skill, knowledge and understanding'.

We can see clearly from Inskipp and Proctor's (1993) ideas that we carry into adulthood the instinctual abilities to receive and explore. A Winnicottian orientation would suggest that in our supervisory interactions as a supervisee, be they okay, clumsy, awkward or distracted, we are enacting our instinctual capacity to receive and explore. This is to regain the self-confidence that we can be the authors of our own good, with this happening with the understanding and responsiveness of others. Effective 'receiving and exploring' by supervisees takes place when there is a belief that such activities are occurring in a relationship of understanding and responsiveness (Astrom et al., 1993; Severinsson, 1995). Effective *object presenting* in clinical supervision is the ability to carry out 'person and task orientated behaviours in an integrated way' (Kermode, 1985). Research literature reviewed supports Winnicott's idea that successful *object presenting* should lead the supervisees to realise a sense of their own ability to reach out and make changes in their world of practice. Attention in clinical supervision to 'what the patient has said and done' (Jones, 1996, p. 292) leads to discovery of 'knowledge embedded in practice' (Hallberg, 1994, p. 51) and 'helps nurses to be more patient centred' (Paunonen, 1991). Other reported changes include increased 'willingness to act, freedom of action' (Paunonen, 1991, p. 983), 'courage, self-assurance, mental strength and a sense of well-being' (Palsson et al., 1994, p. 391) and the ability to 'return to the work of patient care with new/renewed strategies for collaboration' (Ritter *et al.*, 1996, p. 150).

An interesting research finding, given the attention paid to the importance of pace in *object presenting*, is Edberg and Hallberg's (1996, p. 145) report of measurable improvements in nurses' abilities to achieve mutuality with patients. This was demonstrated, following a period of clinical supervision, by the nurses' ability to 'act in the same pace' in their care of patients with dementia, when compared with a control group. It is therefore not surprising for Watkins (1995, p. 572) to observe that a supervisor requires a 'good enough sense of timing'.

Another important dimension of *object presenting* in clinical supervision is the impact of the person who is the supervisor. This has received little attention in nursing literature. It is only Palsson *et al.* (1994) who report different consequences in the work of two clinical supervision groups, which might be explained by the supervisor's 'different personalities and training' (Palsson *et al.*, 1994, p. 392).

Unfortunately, the experience of *object presenting*, which results out of educational or clinical relationships, has not led to a fortuitous state where many nurses have the self-confidence to believe they can reach out and make changes to their world of practice, with the expectation that they will meet with understanding and responsiveness (Chan and Rudman, 1998, Johns 2003). As a generalisation, we are more prone to believe that we cannot make things happen, rather than that we can. The failure of nursing to have a shared voice or conviction about its boundaries makes it difficult to define our core purpose and means we are ever open to redefinition by others. One consequence seems to be that the essential ability of maternal provision to be 'good enough' has been devalued in order to achieve 'throughput', as opposed to care.

Paradoxically the view from my goldfish bowl of clinical supervision reveals a nursing workforce which, while hard pressed at times, is also generally ambitious, well educated, ethically aware, articulate, and clinically advanced. Such practitioners strive to reach understandings of clinical practice, which will enable them to deliver 'good enough' care. The act of clinical supervision provides such nurses with opportunities to explore the intricacies of their practice and by doing so, usually reveals the value of their professional self, their actions, and enhances their belief that they can bring about constructive change.

Conclusion

A theory of maternal provision, as a conceptual framework for clinical supervision in nursing is fraught with potential problems and misunderstandings. This interpretation of Winnicott's ideas might be construed as advocating a paternalistic, as opposed to collegial and collaborative approach. This has not been the intention. Hopefully, it has been shown that, within a facilitating environment, it would possible for there to be appropriate equality and chances for self-direction by the supervisee.

What the framework does suggest is that the supervisor, by virtue of their responsibilities for enabling the growth of another, has to have authority of professional purpose. Their accountability, for creating the handling conditions necessary to maximise the supervisee's inherent capacity for growth, means supervisors must have the freedom to set limits or assert professional boundaries.

It could be argued that such a conceptual framework just replaces an existing paternalistic hegemony with one which is maternalistic. The author's intention, though, was to demonstrate the potential for such a set of ideas to inform the supervisory process, in order that clinical supervision can be a means of liberating the developmental potential of the individual and of the profession.

The concepts of holding, handling and object presenting have been used to illustrate the key functions of clinical supervision. Articulating some of the core elements of each concept in supervisory work has been attempted. An overarching set of purposes for clinical supervision is now suggested. These have to do with:

- creating the conditions for professional attachment and security
- making professional and personal change and adaptation possible
- enabling the supervisee to believe they can be the author of their own professional good.

Using Winnicott (1960)

This framework of meaning is true to the maternal nature of nursing and, at its most basic, is an understandable and coherent nursing explanation of clinical supervision.

References

Abbott, S., Johnson, B., Dawson, L., Hutt, J. and Sealy, A. (2006). 'Introducing clinical supervision for community-based nurses.' *British Journal of Community Nursing* 11(8): 346–8.

Adams, T. (1996). 'A descriptive study of the work of community psychiatric nurses with elderly demented people.' *Journal of Advanced Nursing* 23: 1177–85.

Allen, I. (2001). 'Stress among ward Sisters and Charge Nurses.' Policy Studies Institute (PSI). Available from www.psi.org.uk/news/pressrelease.asp?news_item_id = 17 (Accessed 24 August 2008)

Astrom, G., Furaker, C. and Norberg, A. (1993). 'Nurses' skills in managing ethically difficult care situations: interpretation of nurses' narratives.' *Journal of Advanced Nursing* 21: 1073–80.

Bishop, V. (1998). 'What is going on? Results of a questionnaire.' In *Clinical Supervision in Practice*, ed. V. Bishop. London: Macmillan/NT Research, pp. 22–39.

Bodley, D. E. (1992). 'Clinical supervision in psychiatric nursing: using the process record.' *Nurse Education Today* 12(2): 148–55.

Bowlby, J. (1988). *A Secure Base: Clinical Applications of Attachment Theory.* London: Routledge.

Butterworth, T., Bishop, V. and Carson, J. (1996). 'First steps towards evaluating clinical supervision in nursing and health visiting. Theory, policy and practice development. A review.' *Journal of Clinical Nursing* 5(2): 127–32.

Butterworth, T., Carson, J., White, E., Jeacock. J., Clements, A. and Bishop, V. (1997). *'It is good to talk': An Evaluation of Clinical Supervision and Mentorship in England and Scotland.* Manchester: University of Manchester, School of Nursing and Midwifery.

Chambers, M. and Long, A. (1995). 'Supportive clinical supervision: a crucible for personal and professional change.' *Journal of Psychiatric and Mental Health Nursing* 2(5): 311–16.

Chan, P. and Rudman, M. (1998). 'Paradigms for mental health nursing, fragmentation or integration?' *Journal of Psychiatric and Mental Health Nursing* 5(2): 143–5.

City and Hackney Teaching Primary Care Trust (2006). Clinical Supervision Policy & Guidelines for Registered Nurses & Clinical Support Staff. Ref CL003 July 2006. Available from www.chpct.nhs.uk/trust_documents/doc_click_count.asp?id = 296 (Accessed 22 August 2008)

Dartington, A. (1993). 'Where angels fear to tread: idealism, despondency and inhibition in thought in hospital nursing.' *Winnicott Studies* 7 (Spring): 21–41.

Department of Health (1993). *NHS Management Executive: A Vision for the Future. The Nursing, Midwifery and Health Visiting Contribution to Health and Health Care.* London: Stationery Office.

Dudley, M. and Butterworth, T. (1994). 'The cost and some benefits of clinical supervision: an initial exploration.' *International Journal of Psychiatric Nursing Research* 1(2): 34—40.

Dudley Group of Hospitals (2004). Nursing and Midwifery Strategy. Policy NC24 Clinical Supervision. Available from www.dudley.nhs.uk/sections/publications/documents/FOI24954894933.pdf (Accessed 24 August 2008)

Edberg, A.K. and Hallberg, I.R. (1996). 'Effects of clinical supervision on nurse-patient co-operation quality: a controlled study in dementia care.' *Clinical Nursing Research* 5(2): 127–46.

Fabricius, J. (1991). 'Running on the spot or can nursing really change.' *Psychoanalytic Psychotherapy* 5: 97–108.

Faugier, J. (1992a). 'The supervisory relationship.' In *Clinical Supervision and Mentorship in Nursing*, eds. T. Butterworth and J. Faugier. London: Chapman and Hall, pp.18–36.

Faugier, J. (1992b). *'Casework conversations.'* In *Clinical Supervision and Mentorship in Nursing*, eds. T. Butterworth and J. Faugier. London: Chapman and Hall, pp. 214–29.

Gomez, L. (1997). *An Introduction to Object Relations.* London: Free Association Books.

Hallberg, I.R. and Norberg, A. (1993). 'Strain amongst nurses and their emotional reactions during one year of systematic clinical supervision combined with implementation of individualised care in dementia nursing.' *Journal of Advanced Nursing* 18: 1860–75.

Hallberg, I.R. (1994). 'Systematic clinical supervision in a child psychiatric ward: nursing care, tedium, burnout and the nurses' own report on the effects of it.' *Archives Psychiatric Nursing* 8(1): 44–52.

Hughes, L. and Pengelly, P. (1997). *Staff Supervision in a Turbulent Environment.* London: Jessica Kingsley Publishers.

Inskipp, F. and Proctor, B. (1993). *Making the Most of Supervision (Part 1).* Twickenham: Cascade.

Jansson, L. and Norberg, A. (1993). 'Ethical reasoning among experienced nurses concerning the feeding of terminally ill cancer patients.' *Cancer Nursing* 12(6): 352–8.

Jenkins, E., Parke, S. and Rafferty, M. (2000). 'Clinical supervision: what is happening in West Wales?' *Nursing Times Research* 5(1): 21–37.

Johns, C. (2003). 'Clinical supervision as a model for clinical leadership.' *Journal of Nursing Management* 11(1): 25–35.

Jones, A. (1996). 'Clinical supervision: a framework for practice.' *International Journal of Psychiatric Nursing Research* 3(1): 290–306.

Jones, A. (1997). 'Death, poetry, psychotherapy and clinical supervision (the

contribution of psychodynamic psychotherapy to palliative care nursing).'
Journal of Advanced Nursing 25: 238–44

Kermode, S. (1985). 'Clinical supervision in nurse education: some parallels with teacher education.' *Australian Journal of Advanced Nursing* 2(3): 39–45

Lawler, J. (1991). *Behind the Screens*. Melbourne: Churchill Livingstone.

Leicester County and Rutland NHS Primary Care Trust (2006). Clinical Supervision Policy. Available from
www.lcrpct.nhs.uk/.../Clinical/GeneralPolicies/0/GP003%20Clinical%20Supervision%
(Accessed 24 August 2008)

Marris, P. (1986). *Loss and Change*, 2nd edn. London: Routledge.

McCormack, N. and Hopkins, E. (1995). 'The development of clinical leadership through supported reflective practice.' *Journal of Clinical Nursing* 4(3): 161–8.

McVicar, A. (2003). 'Workplace stress in nursing: a literature review.' *Journal of Advanced Nursing* 44(6): 633–42.

Menzies, I. (1959). 'A case study in the functioning of social systems as a defence against anxiety: a report on a study of the nursing service of a general hospital.' *Human Relations* 13: 95–121.

Mimura, C. and Griffiths, P. (2003). 'The effectiveness of current approaches to workplace stress management in the nursing profession: an evidence based literature review.' *Occupational and Environmental Medicine* 60: 10–15.

Morcom, C. and Hughes, R. (1996). 'How can clinical supervision become a real vision for the future?' *Journal of Psychiatric and Mental Health Nursing* 3(2): 117–24.

Morton-Cooper, A. and Palmer, A. (1993). *Mentorship and Preceptorship*. Oxford: Blackwell Science.

NHS Scotland (2008). Clinical Supervision. Flying start NHS developing confident, capable health practitioners. Available from:
www.flyingstart.scot.nhs.uk/ClinicalSupervision.htm (Accessed 24 August 2008)

Nightingale, F. (1860). *Notes on Nursing: What It Is and What It Is Not*. London: Harrison and Sons.

Nursing Times Magazine (2007). 'Stress "harms nurses' sex lives".'
Available from: http://news.bbc.co.uk/1/hi/health/6691017.stm
(Accessed 28 May 2007)

Nursing and Midwifery Council (2008a). Clinical supervision for registered nurses (updated April 2008).
Available from: http://www.nmc-uk.org./cms/content/advice/clinical
(Accessed 24 August 2008)

Nursing and Midwifery Council (2008b). Modern supervision in action, a practical guide for midwifes (January 2008). Available from: www.midwifery supervision.scot.nhs.uk/publications/Modern_Supervision_in_Action.pdf
(Accessed 24 August 2008)

Palsson, M.B., Hallberg, I.R., Norberg, A. and Isovaara, S. (1994). 'Systematic clinical supervision and its effects for nurses handling demanding care situations: interviews with Swedish district nurses and hospital nurses in cancer care.' *Cancer Nursing* 17: 385–94.

Paunonen, M. (1991). 'Changes initiated by a nursing supervision programme: an analysis based on log-linear models.' *Journal of Advanced Nursing* 16: 982–6.

Peplau, H.E. (1988). *Interpersonal Relations in Nursing*. Houndmills, Hampshire: Macmillan.

Phillips, A. (1988). 'Winnicott.' In *Fontana Modern Masters*, ed. F. Kermode. London: Fontana.

Proctor, B. (1987). 'Supervision: a co-operative exercise in accountability.' In *Enabling and Ensuring: Supervision in Practice*. Leicester: National Youth Bureau and Council for Education and Training in Youth and Community Work.

Rafferty, M. (1998). 'Clinical supervision.' In *Face to Face with Distress*, eds. E. Barnes, P. Griffiths, J. Ord and D.Wells. Oxford: Butterworth Heinemann, pp.188–97.

Rafferty, M. (1999). 'A study of student responses to an educational preparation for clinical supervision.' *WNB Occasional Papers The Development of Professional Practice*, Issue No 3, pp.14–18. Cardiff: The Welsh National Board.

Rafferty, M. and Coleman, M. (1996). 'Educating nurses to undertake clinical supervision in practice.' *Nursing Standard* 10: 38–41.

Rafferty, M., Jenkins, E. and Parke, S. (1998). *Clinical Supervision: What is going on in West Wales?* A Report to the Clinical Effectiveness Unit (Wales), The School of Health Science (University of Wales, Swansea), March.

Rafferty, M., Llewellyn, B. and Hewitt, J. (2007). *Setting Standards for the Practice of Clinical Supervision – A Welsh Perspective. In Practising Clinical Supervision A Reflective Approach* (2nd edn), ed. J. Driscoll. Philadelphia, PA: Elsevier Publishing, pp. 217–41.

Ritter, S., Norman, I., Rentoul, L. and Bodley, D. (1996). 'A model of clinical supervision for nurses undertaking short placements in mental health care settings.' *Journal of Clinical Nursing* 5(3): 149–58.

Royal College of Nursing (RCN) (2008a). *Evidence to the NHS Pay Review Body (2007), Vacancies in NHS England 2007*. Available from www.rcn.org.uk/__data/assets/word_doc/0008/108908/Evidence_to_the_NHS_ Pay_ Review_Body_2008_final.doc. (Accessed 24 August 2008)

Royal College of Nursing (RCN) (2008b). *Nurses' working hours 'too long'*. Available from: news.bbc.co.uk/1/hi/wales/7411785.stm (Accessed 24 August 2008)

Salisbury Health Care Trust (2004). *Clinical Supervision guidelines for practice*. Available from www.salisbury.nhs.uk/.../clinicalsupervision/clinicalsupervision guidelinesforpracticejul04.pdf. (Accessed 24 August 2008)

Severinsson, E. (1995). 'The phenomenon of clinical supervision in psychiatric health care.' *Journal of Psychiatric and Mental Health Nursing* 2: 301–10.

Skogstad, W. (1997). 'Working in a world of bodies: defensive techniques on a medical ward – a psychoanalytical observation.' *Psychoanalytic Psychotherapy* 11: 221–41.

Smith, P. (1992). *The Emotional Labour of Nursing*. Houndmills, Basingstoke: Macmillan.

Snelgrove, S. (1998). 'Occupational stress and job satisfaction: A comparative study of health visitors, district nurses and community psychiatric nurses.' *Journal of Nursing Management* 6: 97–104.

Swain, G. (1995). *Clinical Supervision: The Principles and Process*. London: Health Visitors' Association.

Titchen, A. and Binnie, A. (1995). 'The art of clinical supervision.' *Journal of Clinical Nursing* 4(5): 327–34.

UKCC (United Kingdom Central Council for Nursing, Midwifery and Health Visiting)(1996). *The Position Statement on Clinical Supervision for Nursing and Health Visiting*. London: UKCC.

Watkins, C.E. (1995). 'Psychotherapy supervision in the 1990s: some observations and reflections.' *American Journal of Psychotherapy* 49(4): 568–81.

Winnicott, D.W. (1960). 'The theory of the parent-infant relationship.' *International Journal of Psychoanalysis* 41: 585–95.

Winnicott, D.W. (1988). *Human Nature*. London: Free Association Books.

Winship, G. (1995). 'The unconscious impact of caring for acutely disturbed patients: a perspective for supervision.' Journal of Psychiatric and Mental Health Nursing 2: 227–31.

Winstanley, J. (2001). 'Developing methods for evaluating clinical supervision.' In *Contemporary Themes in Clinical Supervision*, eds. J. Cutcliffe, T. Butterworth and B. Proctor. London: Routledge, pp. 210–24.

Wolsey, P. and Leach, L. (1997). 'Clinical supervision: A hornet's nest?' *Nursing Times* 93(44): 24–7.

Worcestershire NHS Mental Health Partnership (2005). Policy for clinical supervision for nurses. Available from www.worcestershirehealth.nhs.uk/ SWPCT_Library/Policies_and_Procedures/Clinical /ClinicalSupervsionPolicy.pdf (Accessed 23 August 2008)

Yegdich, T. and Cushing, A. (1998). 'An historical perspective on clinical supervision in nursing.' *Australian and New Zealand Journal of Mental Health Nursing* 7: 3–24.

Index